THE
STORIES
WITHIN

THE STORIES WITHIN

Developing inclusive drama and story-making

SHEREE VICKERS and ROSIE EMANUEL

HINTON HOUSE Therapeutic Resources

HINTONHOUSE

Dedication

Sheree: To the All Stars drama group, a wonderful team of dramatic players who inspired and charmed all who met them.

Rosie: To everyone at the Orpheus Centre who have taught me so much. Also to my family, and to Tom, for everything.

First published in 2011 by

Hinton House Publishers Ltd, Newman House, 4 High Street, Buckingham, MK18 1NT, UK

T +44 (0)1280 822557 F +44 (0) 560 3135274 E info@hintonpublishers.co.uk

www.hintonpublishers.co.uk

British Library Cataloguing in Publication Data

Vickers, Sheree.

  The stories within : developing inclusive drama & story-making.

  1. Drama—Study and teaching. 2. Storytelling—Study and teaching.

  3. Drama in education. 4. Storytelling in education. 5. Drama—Therapeutic use.

  6. Narrative therapy.

  I. Title II. Emanuel, Rosie.

  371.3'99-dc22

ISBN 978 1 906531 22 5

Printed and bound in the United Kingdom by Hobbs the Printers Ltd.

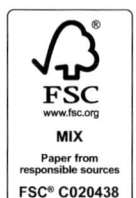

FSC
www.fsc.org
MIX
Paper from responsible sources
FSC® C020438

Contents

PART II DRAMA & STORY STRUCTURES

PART III USING EXISTING STORIES AS A STARTER

Contents

List of Handouts

Acknowledgements

Sarah Watney, for all her help in the development and initial implementation of the 'Romeo & Juliet' workshops.

Jules Oakshett, who co-created and co-led the 'Clue Bags' workshops.

Fran Chabrel and Caroline Segolo, for their work on the 'Dream Catchers' project.

Danny Braverman, for his contributions in the initial thinking stages of the 'Clue Bags' workshops.

Unicorn Theatre for Children for the inclusion of both the 'Blue Fish' and 'AZ & The McPuppets' workshops that were developed as part of the Playbook Project 2005.

Mousetrap Theatre Projects for the inclusion of the 'Clue Bags' workshop, originally developed for the London Theatre Challenge Project, 2007.

Polka Children's Theatre and Merton Music Foundation, for the inclusion of the 'Dream Catchers' workshops, developed in 2007.

A number of these workshops and stories were first published in *Information Exchange*, a multisensory publication for parents and teachers of disabled children.

'Blue Fish' was first published in Issue 68, Spring 2006

'The Disappearing Monkeys' was first published in Issue 75/76, Winter 2008

Finally, a big thank you to all those who have shared their stories with us over the years.

About the Authors

Sheree Vickers is a drama teacher, facilitator, writer and director with nearly 15 years experience in leading groups of all ages and abilities. She has spent a great deal of time working within both the education system and the community developing theatre projects with people who might not always have access to the arts.

As well as being the current Artistic Director at SAVVY Theatre Company, she has also facilitated workshops for London Bubble, Polka Theatre, the Shakespeare Schools Festival, the Soho Theatre Writers Festival, Mousetrap Theatre Projects and was the Education Officer at Unicorn Theatre.

Sheree has written numerous magazine articles and teacher reference materials on her work within the SEN classroom. She is also the author of several books including the Active Drama Playscripts series and *Drama Scripts for People with Special Needs*.

Rosie Emanuel is a Dramatherapist and Drama Practitioner with a range of experience in Special Educational Needs and Disability Arts. She is currently Drama Coordinator at The Orpheus Centre – a performing arts college for young disabled adults in Surrey. As a Dramatherapist she works in the education sector, delivering therapy sessions to children with emotional, behavioural and communication difficulties. She is co-founder of 'The Dramatherapists', a company which offers therapy sessions and training in the field of Dramatherapy.

Since 2003 Rosie has delivered workshops in a variety of settings and contexts for companies such as Polka Children's Theatre, Spare Tyre Theatre Company and Mousetrap Theatre Projects. She also works as a trainer, delivering sessions in Inclusive Drama Practice to teachers and practitioners. Rosie has written a number of Special Educational Needs resource packs and has published articles in both Education and Dramatherapy Journals.

Introduction

We all need to tell our story and to understand our story [...] We need for life to signify, to touch the eternal, to understand the mysterious, to find out who we are.

(Bill Moyers in J. Campbell's *The Power of Myth*)

THE AIM OF THIS BOOK

This practical handbook aims to provide teachers, parents, carers and practitioners with a toolkit for creating original stories with children and adults who have a variety of learning styles and needs. In this resource you will find a range of practical tools, tips and ideas that will boost your confidence and allow your groups to take ownership of their stories, whilst enhancing their (and your) creative capacity. The book may be especially useful for primary and secondary teachers within both SEN and mainstream settings, care workers in care settings such as elderly homes or hospices, creative practitioners, arts therapists, youth workers, and parents/carers of disabled children or adults. Whilst it would not be possible to outline how *every* activity or theme included might be adapted for different groups, the content of this book can be applied to most group settings and circumstances, with people of all ages and needs.

The telling of stories is a vital tradition that allows us to explore who we are and how we are connected with the rest of the world. We all tell and remember stories throughout our lives, whether it is a bedtime ritual associated with childhood, or the recalling of events from the day. By passing on the stories that mean the most to us we feel acknowledged and recognised. Often, we may not feel that a particular event is significant until we share the experience with another. This clarification not only helps us to cement the experience, but also gives us the chance to reflect on and learn from it.

The power of *traditional* story such as myth and fairytale has been universally recognised for many hundreds of years, and the retelling of such tales continues to offer great learning, comfort and inspiration to people of all ages. Yet our focus here is not primarily on traditional story. In this book we are more interested in the 'stories within' that have not yet been told. Perhaps not even complete stories, but the images, symbols and dialogues that come from unconscious places. Through our experience of working professionally in this field, we have come to recognise how valuable and therapeutic it can be for people to bring to life and share their imaginative ideas in a creative and safe space.

This may be especially true when it comes to groups of people who have limited opportunity to express their ideas in a traditional, verbal capacity. What of those whose preference is non-verbal? People who have communication impairments, advanced dementia or complex disabilities, for example, need to be supported and facilitated to share their imaginative ideas in their preferred communication style, whatever that may be. Through this book we aim to explore how this can be made possible and how drama and story-making can be made accessible to all.

Ultimately we hope to encourage and enable you to create drama and stories with your groups, harnessing their individual creativity and finding theatrical ways in which their communication needs can be utilised so that they are able to take ownership of their imaginative journeys. We aim to show how children and adults with *any* communication style can offer valid and meaningful contributions to story-making, if given the opportunity.

IT'S OK TO PLAY

If you're not a workshop leader or drama teacher, the idea of getting up in front of a group of people and acting out characters or telling stories may make you feel uncomfortable. You might be a very creative care worker who would love to find the confidence to lead storytelling sessions, but don't feel you have the strategies or ideas to make it happen.

It is important to trust the fact that play comes naturally to most people if they feel *safe* enough to express themselves freely, without fear of judgement. Drama and storytelling start with play. In order for play to be at the heart of any workshop or classroom experience, the leader of the session needs to be at ease both within themselves and the space they are working in. The aim for anyone leading a session is to encourage everyone to share in 'collective play'.

Playing is the most natural thing in the world for a child to do; through play a child discovers how the world works and their place within it. But for adults, playing can feel less natural. Generally, adults tend to only allow themselves to play within strict rule-based games such as sports, which have little freedom for imaginative input. Often, there is also stigma attached to the idea of playing in our work-focused society, where play and leisure can be seen as luxury rather than necessity. We may also feel foolish when asked to participate in a playful activity. By adolescence we have developed a much stronger awareness of how we are perceived by others and how we want to be perceived. Playfulness involves an element of risk, and some may find that the risk, for them, is too great.

When contemplating leading a storytelling session, it is important that you feel comfortable to encourage and *model* playfulness. This is not only for the participants but also for other staff who may be working alongside you. If you're new to leading drama or storytelling sessions and are worried about how the other staff will respond, try setting up a session with just those staff members before you begin working with the group. Explain what you are aiming to achieve within the session, introduce and demonstrate some of the activities you are going to use and encourage feedback. Who knows, they might have some ideas themselves on how the session could work. Encouraging support staff to be involved in the process can help all involved to lose their inhibitions. You may find that the group responds much more readily to the sessions if all the staff present are comfortable with the idea of playing.

Another worry that can occur is the fear of not having ideas, or of not being 'creative enough' to come up with a story. Again, the story-leader is not expected to create the entire story themselves, but is there to set up a structure in which a story can develop in any number of ways. Nor are we asking those new to the process of story-making to work far outside their comfort zone.

Storytelling and drama should be fun, and the exhilaration comes through the challenges and surprises that can occur within each session. Provided the environment feels safe, then stories and ideas should start to flow naturally. Even if they don't, it is fine to admit to this; no-one is supposed to have all the answers! Often, admitting that you don't know where the story should go next can draw out even more imaginative ideas from the group, leading to fascinating results.

This book is all about encouraging story-leaders to have a go and *take a risk*. There is always going to be an element of unpredictability about story-making – of delving deep into the 'unknown' – but it is this unknown element which makes the work exciting and potentially therapeutic. Ultimately it is about trusting that your group *will tell the stories that they need and want to tell*. Our job is to facilitate this process. Through the following chapters our aim is to equip you with solid workshop structures, drama strategies, games and tips, giving you a safety net that will help you to feel more able to take risks and begin your journey into the unknown with confidence and vigour.

THE DRAMATHERAPY QUESTION

In order to thoroughly understand the context of this book, it seems important to make a clear distinction between what is described here and the practice of *Dramatherapy*. The workshops and projects described in this book are for use by professionals who may not have any therapeutic training (teachers, practitioners, youth workers, care workers, parents) and therefore what is described here should not be seen as an intentional therapeutic intervention.

The British Association of Dramatherapists (BADth) defines Dramatherapy as 'the intentional use of the healing aspects of drama and theatre within the therapeutic process'. Dramatherapists therefore have a clear aim to facilitate personal insight, growth and change by working with unconscious processes through drama, play and creative interaction. The therapist may work consistently with a client over a number of months or years, building a strong therapeutic relationship and working confidentially in a contained and private space. It is a practice that is focused on the health and emotional well-being of clients, and Dramatherapists are therefore trained and registered as Health Professionals with the Health Professions Council (HPC).

When working with drama and story-making the aims of the work might be to:

★ Develop social, communication or independence skills

★ Build confidence and self-esteem

★ Work as a team

★ Allow each person's voice to be heard

★ Offer opportunities to explore and enhance the imagination

★ Develop playfulness and creativity

★ Explore aspects of the curriculum in a way that caters for preferred learning styles

★ Develop a piece of theatre or an original story

This is not to say that working with material such as that described in this book will not have therapeutic benefits; if facilitated effectively there is every chance that it will. However, this therapeutic value will be *symptomatic* of participation in the creative work, and is therefore not a specific aim but a likely outcome.

IS THE ELEMENT OF PERFORMANCE IMPORTANT?

Throughout this book we state that groups (and practitioners) should not always be encouraged to 'perform', as the element of performance in drama can lead to anxiety about getting it right. Yet there can also be benefits when people work towards a performance; it can aid in their commitment to a project and provide a sense of achievement and closure.

Therefore, it is important to explore exactly what a 'performance' is and its relevance to your group. Many groups feel the need to share their work with an audience and this is important. Even those who do not want to perform for an outside audience (such as family, friends or invited guests) may still want to show their work to others within the group.

Using the term 'sharing' can also take the pressure off any individuals who might not want to perform, and any facilitators who feel that they might be expected to mount a major production.

In this context, the aim of putting on any performance is about letting the audience get a glimpse of the special work produced during the workshop or project. For those involved in the actual show, it is not about training participants to be professional actors but rather encouraging them to have a professional attitude towards the work that they produce.

SOME KEY POINTS ON INCLUSIVE PRACTICE

Inclusive practice has become increasingly relevant in all types of groupwork over the past few years. Many schools, institutions and extra-curricular activities are exploring what being 'inclusive' means to them. This book is not about dictating what your inclusion policy should be, nor is it about creating a definition of the term. Yet through the projects we have been involved with, numerous questions and discussions have arisen around inclusive practice, leading to some useful findings. The following key points have guided our practice.

Tips for Inclusive Practice

★ **Ensure you have adequate support**

To fully involve a group with diverse support and communication needs in drama work, additional staff training or adequate one-to-one support might be required.

★ **Get to know individual needs**

By assessing communication and access needs in advance, you will have a greater chance of keeping the participants engaged, focused and excited by the work throughout.

★ **Evaluate each session and make adjustments accordingly**

For example, there might be someone who is constantly causing a disruption, so different strategies may be needed to help include that person.

★ **Consider the group set up**

For example, for maximum participation would shorter sessions with smaller groups work better than having everyone together for the entire session? An 'all-inclusive' policy does not necessarily mean having everyone all together throughout.

★ **Monitor group dynamics**

This can be particularly important if introducing someone new into a group.

★ **Closely monitor your policies**

Have an open approach to any inclusion policy by keeping the debate open as to what inclusivity means for your group.

PART I

Practicalities

GETTING STARTED

Props & Materials

Before you begin creating plans and outlines for your drama or story-making work, it's essential to think through the practical side of things. If you don't have access to a good range of sensory materials then you may want to collect some beforehand, in order that they are accessible whenever you need them. Sensory props and materials are at the heart of all the workshops described in this book, as our experience has shown us that those with sensory or communication impairments in particular are able to access the work much more readily when there is something tangible and physical for them to explore.

Each project in the 'Drama & Story Structures' section has its own list of specific materials needed for each activity, but what follows is a list of sensory materials that we have found especially useful for general story-making with people who have particular communication and/or learning needs.

The Space

Preparation

Getting the space right can make all the difference to the success of the session or workshop, yet this can often be the most difficult element to achieve. Often the space in which we work is beyond our control. For instance, in a school the session may have to be run in a classroom full of tables, chairs and a variety of distractions. To avoid such a scenario it is important to do your research. If at all possible try

Ingredients for a Sensory Storytelling Kit

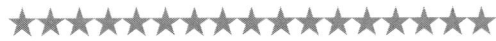

★★★★★★★★★★★★★★★★★★

HANDOUT 1

★ A sensory ball or two (e.g., soft, spiky, lights up, big enough to hold easily).

★ A range of percussion instruments that are easy to grasp, e.g., shakers.

★ A medium-sized, good quality drum (such as a djembe).

★ A range of material/fabric in various textures and colours including:

- lycra for stretching;

- shimmering blue material to represent sea or sky;

- ribbons or scarves in a range of colours.

★ A variety of animal puppets, both land and sea animals.

★ Natural objects such as shells, stones, fossils, wood, pine cones.

★ Water spray bottles (empty spray bottles are available in any mainstream pharmacy store).

★ A small range of scented oils such as lavender, citrus and spices.

★ A few fans to create a breeze or strong wind.

★ Non-toxic drawing materials including marker pens and large sheets of paper.

★ A music player and a selection of different music styles.

to visit and see the space beforehand so that you can get an idea of what you're working with. If you aren't able to see the space then make sure that someone describes it to you, to give you an idea of its size and layout. If you are a visiting practitioner then ask the relevant teacher to prepare the space before you arrive, telling them how you want it to look. If you're working in a classroom then try to ensure that tables are moved to the sides of the room before you arrive and that there is space to move around freely where possible.

Size

The size of the space will have a direct impact on the work you are trying to achieve. If it is too small then you will need to make your storytelling or drama less movement-based and more led by images and objects. If the space is huge then you may want to mark out a smaller space with masking tape on the floor (or with benches), as a space that is too large can be intimidating and it can be more challenging to keep participants focused. Some people with disabilities such as those on the autism spectrum can be hugely affected by the space, especially if it is a space that is new to them. For longer-term projects it is important to ensure that you can have the same space for every session. A change in the space half-way through a project can be very difficult for some people with special needs to tolerate, and this might prevent them from being able to access the sessions.

Privacy

If working with a group over a period of time, then ideally the work should take place in a space that can be made private. Interruptions can have an impact on the group's willingness to take risks and offer ideas to the sessions and it can also be very distracting. When exploring the world of the imagination we are asking people to share part of their internal world and this involves an element of risk. If the space in which we facilitate this work does not feel safe, then the group is unlikely to feel free enough to explore and express their ideas. If the group feels that the space in which they are working is safe and containing, then they should feel more able to share and offer ideas to the creative work.

Creating a Welcoming Space

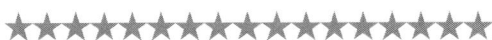

★★★★★★★★★★★★★★★★★★★★★

★ If the space is cluttered with items not relevant to your session then use some large sheets of fabric, such as muslin, to cover everything irrelevant. If these pieces of fabric are different colours this can create an inviting and more neutral space for the participants to enter, and it also means that there is less opportunity for distraction.

★ Play a CD of relaxing music as the participants enter, or play music appropriate to the theme of the session.

★ Drip lavender oil onto the radiators or use a room-spray before the group enters. This can also be used to add a sensory element to the story-making, such as smelling the lavender oil when imagining 'walking across the heaths and hills'.

★ If people can see into the room through doors or windows, hang some material over these to stop onlookers from gazing in and making the group feel like 'performers' with an audience. It will also stop the group from being distracted by what is going on outside.

★ If you feel it may be necessary, place a 'Please Do Not Disturb' sign on the door.

★ When working with young people, try using coloured mats or small squares of material so that each person has their own 'space' to which they can return whenever necessary. This can be very containing for children with special needs and allows them to feel that they have their own place within the larger space, should they want to draw back from the groupwork. You can introduce this concept very early on as a game, for example, "When the music stops, everyone return to your mat!" (If you have a good amount of time with the group, the first sessions could be spent making their own individual mats, using fabric paints, for example).

Creating a Welcoming Space

Working with vulnerable people means that consistency can make all the difference in their ability to feel secure enough to participate fully. Realistically, these elements are not easy to put in place and so you may find yourself having to be imaginative in order to make a space more workable. If the space is inviting from the moment the participants enter, then you will be off to a good start. You want to draw the group in, and the suggested tips can help make the space more welcoming.

It may be that the space you are using is very familiar to the group you are working with and so it can often help to transform it into somewhere new and exciting for the story-making session. Similarly, if you are a parent of a disabled child or young person and you want to try story-making at home, work with your child to transform the room into a storytelling space. This can become part of the story-making ritual, for example, before you begin the story you can transform it into a 'story land' and at the end return from story land by removing the materials and placing them back into a 'story basket'. This can help the child to differentiate between reality and the imagined world of the story, bringing them clearly back into the 'here and now'.

Entering the Space

Once your space is ready, think about how you want the group to enter. Do you want them to enter individually or as a whole? If you choose to have them enter the space as a group, you could try a number of different strategies. The ideas in Handout 3 may help with any behavioural challenges but could also become part of an opening and closing ritual.

Even if you want group members to come in one by one, it is always best to try and have the entire group ready to enter at the start of the session, as this adds to the anticipation and enhances the sense of ritual. However, sometimes you may find that the session needs to begin even though you are waiting for latecomers. Rather than starting the session late or interrupting a group activity mid-way in order to incorporate latecomers, set up an activity that will keep the group busy while also introducing individuals into the main story-making space. This activity can then

Ideas for Entering the Story Space

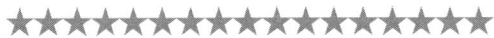

★★★★★★★★★★★★★★★★★★★

★ Lead the group in single file singing a welcome song or chant. Younger children may enjoy marching or doing a series of 'Follow-the-Leader' movements. Each week a different child could lead the group into the session.

★ Invite the group to enter the space by all holding onto a rope to keep everyone together. This is especially effective if working with people with sight-impairments and also acts as a ritual 'joining' of the group from the outset.

★ Create a tunnel using tables covered in cloths that the group has to crawl through to enter the room. If working with those with physical disabilities, support staff could hold a long piece of material above their heads to make a high tunnel, allowing everyone to enter easily.

★ Create a series of stepping-stones leading up to the room, or trails of intriguing objects for the group to collect like a treasure hunt (ideally linked to the theme of the session).

★ Make an interesting 'doorway' for the group to pass through, such as shimmering fabric, bubbles or hanging ribbons. This would also work well with adult groups.

occupy latecomers until an appropriate moment is found to incorporate them into the story-making process.

Introductory Activities

★ Lay a large sheet of paper (the back of a roll of wallpaper always works well) across the room and invite everyone to draw something linked to the theme of the session, or a memory from last week. Another idea is to draw around the group's hands or feet as a symbol of their presence in the room. You could then use this piece of art as a backdrop for the storytelling sessions each week.

★ Set up an opening ritual whereby each person sticks a paper leaf onto a paper tree to represent their presence as they enter the room. By the end of the project you should have a tree covered in leaves. This would also be a good ending ritual, as each participant could draw a picture or write a word on a leaf to represent something they want to remember from the story told that day. By the end you will have a great visual representation of the journey everyone has been on.

★ If working with older adults, particularly those with dementia, it often helps to create a space that contains something immediately familiar and inviting. This might be as simple as serving tea and biscuits at the start of every session so that the group has something to do as soon as they enter the room. Drinking tea is also a symbol of socialising and relaxation and could prevent the participants feeling anxious about the unknown element of the session (for further tips see 'Working with Adults', p. 31).

As explained earlier, if you can manage to provide the group with a creative and user-friendly space for story-making then you're off to a good start. The introduction to each of the 'Drama & Story Structures' contains notes on how the space was managed for each of the projects, which may give you further thoughts and ideas on how to set up your own space.

Group Size

There is no definitive answer to the question of what makes an ideal group size as it is completely dependent on the needs of each group. However, the numbers present will affect the group dynamic significantly. Sometimes a small group can be intimidating for some participants as they can feel that there is too much focus on them individually, while groups that are too large can be difficult to manage when it comes to ensuring that everyone's voice is heard. Those with more complex needs will ideally work in a smaller group and have one-to-one support where necessary, whereas a group with fewer needs is likely to be able to work in larger numbers with less support.

Support Staff

If you are working with unfamiliar participants, you will need to allow time for trust to develop between you and the group. When it comes to support, communication really is the key to success. As the group leader or facilitator, it is your job to ensure that any support staff know the aims of the session and understand the best way of supporting individuals within the group. The most interesting stories will be created in an environment where the support workers understand their role and what is expected of them.

To help facilitate this you may need to meet with support staff before the session begins to run through who they will be working with. If you are lucky enough to have consistent support each week then it can be best to assign the same person to any member of the group who needs one-to-one support, so that a trusting relationship can be built. If you are working in an environment where you don't have (or need) one-to-one support, then allow staff to judge for themselves where support is needed as the session evolves. Either way, the quality of support can make all the difference to the group's (and your) enjoyment of the story-making process.

Regardless of their level of involvement, it is vital that support workers act as 'role models' in the creative process. Should the group get stuck or if no ideas are flowing, support staff can step in and offer examples or ideas to help get the ball rolling again, without taking over the process. They can also encourage participation by working directly with a youngster during an activity. For example, a support worker might go 'under the sea' (moving under some blue material) *with* a participant initially, to give them the confidence that it is fun and safe to do so. The next time this activity occurs you may find that the group member is able to join in without prompting or support. Good support workers should be able to judge when to offer assistance and when to give someone space. There is huge potential in these creative activities for individuals to develop their confidence and independence skills if they are supported sensitively.

Parents & Carers

If you are working on a project where parents or carers are directly involved in supporting their child then you may want to approach things differently. Running storytelling sessions with children and their parents/carers can be an extremely valuable way of encouraging creative play and interaction. It can sometimes be challenging for parents or carers to have to try and think of new and interesting ways to play with their child, so by participating in a session led by a professional, they will have the opportunity to interact creatively without the pressure of having to be endlessly creative. If you're a practitioner running interactive family sessions then it is just as important to ensure that the parents/carers understand what is expected of them during the process, as it is with your professional support workers.

The introduction to 'The Sleeping Boy' project describes our experience of incorporating parents into story sessions and how crucial it is to be clear from the outset whether parents are there as participants or observers. A mixture of the two is not ideal, as those parents who do participate may then feel uncomfortable with being watched by other adults. Consequently, this could have an impact on the child's willingness to participate and may create a difficult dynamic to facilitate. Ensuring that everyone present in the storytelling space is there to participate will encourage a more free and natural story-making process, enhancing the experience for everyone involved.

Unwilling Staff/Helpers

The main issue in terms of support is to ensure *commitment* from whoever undertakes this role. Whether the support comes from professionals, parents, carers or siblings, what is needed is a respect for the work and a commitment to participate in the process, without judgement or prejudice. There are times when a teacher might see a visiting drama workshop as an opportunity to withdraw and get on with some marking. This is an understandable desire but also not acceptable if you are relying on them for support. Don't be afraid to confront someone if they are not offering you the support that you need, or are trying to dominate a session with their own ideas. However, if you are clear from the outset about what you need, this problem shouldn't arise. By communicating clearly your needs and expectations from the support staff or parents, you will ensure that the group is given the best opportunity to express their ideas and have their voices heard.

PREPARATION & PLANNING

Knowing Your Group

Knowing your group is an important first step in the preparation process. You may be very familiar with your group, in which case you have an advantage. Knowing the group will allow you to plan a session with the specific individual needs of the group in mind and to arrange the relevant support in advance. On the other hand you may be a facilitator going into a setting 'cold'. This is a tough job but not uncommon for professional practitioners. If you are in this position then ensure that you communicate beforehand with someone who does know the group and get a summary of the group's needs. Remember too, to clarify with the staff member how many will be present in the room and be clear about your maximum group size.

Session Plans & Aims

When it comes to putting together a session plan, everyone has their own style. How much you plan in advance really depends on your level of confidence, your personality and your facilitation style, but having a plan is *always* a good idea even if you only use it as back up. A plan acts like scaffolding for the session. It gives you a structure within which you can then be free. Without a structure, freedom can become chaotic and you can end up losing control. Having a plan in the back of your mind should give you the confidence to allow the session to move in its own direction, knowing that the framework is there to hold the session together if necessary. Some facilitators or teachers like to have the plan to hand for quick reference.

When planning, it is important to consider the *aims* of the session carefully. If your session is a one-off, what is it that you want to achieve by the end of the workshop? Is it simply to have fun or are you looking to encourage teamwork? If you are running a longer-term project then the aims of each session will be different but should still reflect the project's overall goal.

The type of session plan in Handouts 4 and 5 may not suit everyone, but there is clearly room for adaptation and contributions from the group within each section. It is a simple structure that offers space for the group to share their imaginative ideas and have their voices heard. This may be especially important in the first few sessions as the group get to know each other. Once the group is a little more established you may find you are able to make the structure of the session even more flexible.

Sample Workshop Plan

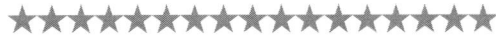

★★★★★★★★★★★★★★★★★★★★

Group Size: 12   Ages of Participants: 12 to 15 years   Session Length: 45 minutes

Range of Needs: Autism spectrum, some wheelchair-users, limited verbal communication

Session Aims

★ To introduce the story of Jack & The Beanstalk

★ To explore physical movement

★ To encourage teamwork

Potential Drama Strategies & Ideas

★ Still images

★ Looking at photographs

★ Use of music and dance

★ Narrative

★ Puppets

Opening Game or Ritual

Physical Name Game – encourage each person to put a movement to the sounds in their name that can then copied by the rest of the group.

Main Workshop

1. Introduce the character of Jack through boy puppet. He introduces the story by showing the group his magic beans.

2. Speculate with the group about what magic the beans might contain. Show Jack's excitement through all of this.

3. Bury the beans in the sand. Develop a gardening movement and/or song with the group.

4. Yawn, stretch and invite group to pretend to sleep. Some dramatic play with Jack puppet, waking up to check on the beans.

5. Music playing as the beanstalk grows. Use long ribbons to brush past the group. Possibly create a dance with ribbons.

6. Place the ribbons around the room and get the group to prepare for their climb up the beanstalk. Journey preparation could involve:

- Inviting group to sit in a circle.
- Get everyone to create an imaginary bag or backpack, sharing the colour or shape of their bag.
- Allow each person to share something they want to take on a journey, either practical (rope, food, matches), fictitious (magic dust, invisible cloak, wise animal) or personal (photos, letters, keepsake).
- Place each item into the bag, marking it with a sound on a musical instrument or asking them to 'Ziiiiip!' up their bag (with whole group joining in).
- 'Pack' each bag and put bags onto backs in preparation for going outdoors (acting out dressing up in imaginary outdoor clothes, taking ideas from group).

N.B. Make a note of the group's ideas of what to take on the journey, as they may become relevant later in the story-making process, such as using a rope to overcome an obstacle.

Closing Game or Ritual

Revisit name game, introducing a 'big' and 'small' element by having the group crouch down and jump up on their names, to reinforce the growing of the beanstalk.

Aims & Ideas for the Next Session

★ Recap beanstalk growing and their journey preparations
★ Pretend to climb up the beanstalk
★ Discover the Giant's house and possible jobs for each servant (exaggerated movements due to the size of the giant)

To Bring

★ Boy puppet
★ Some beans
★ A container with some 'sand'
★ A collection of long green, brown and blue ribbons attached to bamboo poles
★ Music, player and/or some instruments
★ A bag for the journey (optional)

Workshop Plan

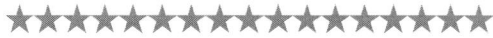

★★★★★★★★★★★★★★★★★★

Group Size: _____ Ages of Participants: _____ Session Length: _____

Range of Needs: _____

Session Aims

★ _____

★ _____

★ _____

Potential Drama Strategies & Ideas

★ _____

★ _____

★ _____

★ _____

★ _____

★ _____

Opening Game or Ritual

_____

_____

Main Workshop

_____

_____

_____

_____

_____

_____

_____

_____

_____

_____

_____
_____
_____
_____
_____
_____
_____
_____
_____
_____
_____
_____
_____

Closing Game or Ritual

_____
_____

Aims & Ideas for the Next Session

★ _____
★ _____
★ _____
_____

To Bring

★ _____
★ _____
★ _____
★ _____
★ _____
★ _____

Themes & Starting Points

Once you know what you want to achieve you can focus the workshop plan in order to achieve this, using appropriate drama ideas to support your aims and explore your theme. If a theme or subject is not specified then often the best place to start is to choose an *environment* as a starting point for the drama. Once the story has an initial environment it gives it a context and stimulates further ideas. You can create soundscapes, draw images or create tableaux of what the environment looks or sounds like and discover who or what lives there. It can also be useful to keep in mind that a successful story can involve:

★ Characters interacting with a setting or environment;

★ A problem or challenge to be overcome;

★ Mystery, adventure, obstacles and conflict;

★ The discovery of assistance to solve a problem;

★ A resolution or ending (which may or may not be positive).

It may be that all you need to get started is an image or object. Images of environments or objects that appear old or valuable make great starting points. For example, a collection of abandoned objects collected from a beach could stimulate questions such as, "Where have the objects come from and how long have they been there?" Perhaps it is the group's job to reunite the objects with their former owners or make a survey for a local environmental agency.

Usually groups will rely on you to provide them with a starting point, which then forms the framework for their ideas. Coming up with a theme or starting point does not mean that you're removing their ownership of the story; you are simply offering them a way in.

Depending on the time available, remember that you don't need to dive straight into the storytelling. If possible, take some time to bring the group together using simple games and exercises. Ball games or percussion circles are very effective ways of creating a sense of cohesion and trust within a group and can also create strong opening and closing rituals (see p. 26 for more detail on Ritual & Repetition). Anything that encourages the group to interact, laugh and make eye-contact will help to put them at ease.

> ## Opening Activity: Lycra Soft Ball
>
> In a seated or standing circle, ask the group to stretch a piece of lycra out across the circle to create a 'platform'. Everyone should be holding onto the edge of the lycra with both hands. The aim of the game is to see how long the group can keep a soft ball rolling on top of the lycra platform, without it falling off the edge!
>
> The lycra can also act as a trampoline to throw the ball up into the air (or you could place a number of soft objects on the surface to make it more difficult).
>
> This game is a fantastic ice-breaker as it is extremely playful and requires good teamwork. Reassure the group that it doesn't matter if the ball falls off the edge, as this is part of the fun.

Session Length

Usually you will have an idea about the length of time available for your session or workshop and can plan accordingly. If you have input into the timing of the session then think about it carefully with your specific group in mind. If you will be leading regular weekly workshops, then around an hour-and-a-half is about right, although this may be too short if the group is quite large and therefore two hours may be better. Often one hour is not enough; you may end up rushing through things and won't have enough time for opening and closing rituals, which are important. It very much depends on the group and you may find that you need to adjust the timing after one or two sessions. Once you know the group a little better you should be able to assess whether the session length is right or needs to be adjusted. If you do need to make any adjustments then do so early on in the process as change can have an impact on a group's sense of safety, especially if working with people on the autism spectrum.

It can be useful to add on an extra 15 minutes at the start to account for latecomers. The first 15 minutes could be a casual, social activity where people can interact more freely (this could involve background music, an art or craft activity, tea or coffee, or songs). This will allow latecomers to enter the space without feeling embarrassed by their lateness. It can be helpful to make a rule whereby latecomers cannot enter after the first half-hour (or 20 minutes for a one-hour session). Having people enter in dribs and drabs can be very disruptive and break the flow of the session, so encourage people to be on time as much as possible. Once you've started the story-making process you need to keep the session as closed and private as possible.

Breaks

Breaks can sometimes be useful and other times quite detrimental. Unfortunately, this might to be something that you have to trial as you get to know the group. A break in the process can be very positive: it can give the group social time to interact more freely, allow them some time out to relax and have a drink, and give you time to take stock of where the story or session is going. On the other hand, a break may cause the group to lose focus or become chaotic and disruptive. If this happens in the first session then you may decide to try it without a break the following week (and perhaps shorten the session time as a result). If you are in an environment where a break is out of your control, then adding a structure to it can help. For example, sit the group down while serving the drinks or snacks and encourage them to take part in with an activity such as drawing images of the story so far. Most people see a break as unstructured time which can be challenging and unsettling for those with additional needs, so it can be beneficial to offer a structured activity within a break if you feel this would help your particular group.

RITUAL & REPETITION

Whatever the age, needs or size of your group, it is important to bear ritual and repetition in mind if you are working with them regularly. There can be an element of risk involved in drama and story-making, as people are asked to express ideas and feelings that are personal and meaningful to them. The group therefore needs to feel that the sessions have structure and are ultimately *contained*. Containment is established not only through the formation of a safe, non-judgemental space, but also through ritual and structure. By creating rituals that can be repeated at each session, familiarity and consistency are provided from week to week. When working with people who have more complex disabilities, repetition can help to reinforce and familiarise, acting as a reminder of previous sessions.

Ritual in storytelling sessions is not about something spiritual or mysterious, but is simply a way of providing your sessions with solid structure, containment and meaning. When working with vulnerable people, this can offer them the security they need in order to feel safe enough to share their ideas and make their voices heard.

Opening Ritual

Circle

Circles are the most natural and easy way to bring a group together, as everyone can see each other and begin on an equal footing. If you have wheelchair-users in the group then invite everyone to sit on chairs so that they are all on the same level. Alternatively some wheelchair-users might prefer to be out of their chairs on the floor. This can be beneficial for some, but does require careful risk assessment and support from people who know the needs of each participant well (e.g., a parent or carer).

Welcome Activity

Once in a circle the opening ritual can be a welcome song, call and response (with voices and/or rhythm), percussion circle or simple name game. Afterwards you may play a few games or exercises relating to the theme or story, which can differ from week to week. However, it can be useful if *the welcome activity is the same each week*. It is the repetition of this activity that offers that all-important containment at the start of each session.

The purpose of the opening ritual is to:

★ Bring the group together and encourage awareness of who is in the room;

★ Make each participant feel that their presence is recognised;

★ Provide familiarity and containment at the start of the session;

★ Harness and focus the group's energy for the upcoming workshop.

Using Names

Welcoming everyone individually by name is critical as a way of acknowledging each person's presence. If some group members are not present, it is good practice to mention their absence. You might say something along the lines of: "Toby and Jess aren't with us today, but we look forward to welcoming them back soon". This will emphasise to the group that everyone is important and that no-one will be forgotten from week to week.

Main Drama or Story Event

Once you feel the group is ready, start the storytelling or drama work after the opening ritual and games. You may want to recap events from the previous week while still in the circle; asking the group to remind you of what happened is a good way of ascertaining what was important and memorable for them. Depending on the group, it can be helpful if there is a transition at this point into the 'world of the story'. This might involve preparation and a journey to get there, perhaps with follow-the-leader style movements or travelling through different landscapes. This transition helps to separate the world of the story and reality. Travelling to and from the story world can add a strong sense of ritual to the session, but remember that if you travel there, you should leave time to travel back!

Often the main part of the session will involve moving in and around the space, depending on the participants' mobility. Breaking out of the circle to continue the storytelling will give the opening and closing circles greater meaning. Movement also helps to keep people energised, especially for those who are kinaesthetic learners and find it difficult to sit and listen for any length of time.

Story Ending

Stop your storytelling at least ten minutes before the end of the session, as the group may need time to be brought back to reality. You could ask them to make a series of still images or tableaux to represent the point the story has reached and take imaginary photographs of the images (or you could take real photos if you have permission). The next session could then start with recreating these images as a reminder of where the story ended.

De-Role & Closing Ritual

Bringing the participants out of character and back to being 'themselves' can sometimes be challenging if they are enjoying their role in the story. The following techniques can help to de-role a group:

★ Invite participants to remove their imaginary costume or to 'shake off' their character. This can be very physical and people can assist each other. As the facilitator you can emphasise the departure of the characters by saying goodbye to them and welcoming each person by name back into the room.

★ When removing the character's imaginary costume, you could ask the group to use some magic to shrink their costume until it is tiny enough to fit into their (or your) pocket until next time.

★ Alternatively, roll the imaginary costumes or even characters into some fabric so that the world of the story is captured safely, ready to be released again the following week.

This kind of physical and visual de-role is especially important for those who find it more difficult to comprehend what is real and what is imaginary. Despite your best efforts there may be times when the de-role process becomes a huge challenge owing to participants assuming characters too deeply. In these cases, having support staff who understand the needs of the group is very important, especially when leading a one-off session.

> ## CASE STUDY
>
> In one school workshop, a boy on the autism spectrum was desperate to play the dragon in the story. It quickly became apparent that he had moved deeply into character, showing little awareness of others in the room. The depth to which he travelled into character was such that all usual methods of 'de-roling' and grounding failed to work. He became very distressed (while still roaring and flying around as the dragon) and it became necessary for him to be taken out of the session by his teacher, in order to give him space to calm down and de-role privately with a familiar person. This was a situation that could not have been predicted but the support from the teacher was critical in order that the situation did not get out of hand.

Closing Activity

Once the de-role is complete, come back into a circle for the closing ritual. Following are a variety of examples of effective closing activities:

★ Allow each person to take a turn banging on a drum, this acts as a strong grounding activity.

★ Stamping is also an effective way to ground those who may be finding it difficult to make the transition out of the imaginary world and back into the here and now.

★ Play a game where participants must touch different parts of the room, for example, such as 'something cold' or 'something red'. Any activity involving making contact with something solid in the room can help to bring people back.

★ Sing a gentle song which everyone can join in, perhaps a 'goodbye' version of your opening ritual.

Whatever you choose for your ending ritual, the most important thing is to repeat it each time the group meets. The repetition of this activity will become symbolic of the session ending and will help the group to recognise this fact.

Ending Celebration

If you are working with a group for a number of weeks or months, it is a good idea to mark the ending of the whole process with some kind of celebration. You may decide to enact your whole story again, with you as narrator and each person choosing a part to play, so the group can experience the story they have created in its complete form. Alternatively, you could set up an art activity where the group creates drawings of the story to make into a storyboard, which can then be displayed. Group members could receive a certificate to mark their contribution to the story and these could be handed out in a special ceremony with you adding a personal comment or reflection about each person.

WORKING WITH ADULTS

Working with adults in a drama or storytelling situation is often no different from working with children and young people; it is still fundamentally about *playing* and drawing out ideas from the group. All of the same key factors apply: creating a safe and creative space, getting the right support, and planning ahead. It would be misleading to suggest that you have to apply a completely different set of skills and techniques when working with adults – you don't. And yet it is worth thinking about any small differences between working with children and adults in this kind of work, so that there are fewer surprises when you get into the room.

Drama and storytelling can be particularly beneficial for adult groups such as those with advanced or onset dementia, suffering from terminal or psychiatric illness, and adults with learning disabilities. Engaging with storytelling can offer a place for the expression of thoughts and feelings indirectly and symbolically, without having to rely on conscious thought. It can be difficult for some people, especially those who rely on non-verbal communication, to find ways of expressing themselves. Drama and storytelling can provide such an opportunity if well-facilitated.

Sessions with adult groups can be exciting and fulfilling, perhaps because adults tend to have fewer opportunities to participate in creative and playful work.

Offering adults a chance to revisit their playful and childish past can be extremely releasing and therapeutic. One of the biggest differences you may come across when working with adult groups is that it can take longer to facilitate playfulness. There may be more resistance to taking risks and can be stronger barriers to participating in something new and unfamiliar. It is critical with any group, but especially when working with adults, to help them to feel at ease from the very beginning. Music is a powerful tool to help people feel more relaxed, as entering a silent room can be intimidating. You could also place some interesting objects or images in the centre of the room on a table or cloth, which act as good conversation starters and give people a common interest within the space. These objects may then be used as starting points for the stories or drama in the rest of the session.

Opening & Closing

The opening ritual is just as important when working with adult groups, although the activity obviously needs to be age-appropriate. Ensure that the song or activity you choose does not patronise the group or make them feel as though they are being treated as children. For a group with dementia, you could create your opening ritual by asking the group about their favourite songs. You can then learn these as a group and sing each song together in a circle (holding hands if appropriate). If your group doesn't have any ideas for songs they like, then you could choose a song and teach it to them. A good ending ritual might be to invite people to move to some favourite music before leaving the room.

Movement & Mobility

If you are working with older adults or those with limited mobility, don't be afraid to encourage physical activity by inviting everyone to participate in any way that they feel comfortable with. Groups of older adults may feel that they are more frail than they actually are (often due to lack of activity), but may soon pick up on the energy of the session and, with encouragement, feel inspired to have a go. Don't underestimate how infectious your enthusiasm and energy can be, although it is important not to push anyone into doing something they are not comfortable with.

Remember too that you don't need to perform to the group to get them energised. You will quickly lose a group's attention if they feel that you are not being real and are trying to put on a show. It can be easy to feel you have to *entertain* your group constantly, especially one which has low energy itself. Find the balance between inspiring the participants with your own energy while still being yourself.

If mobility is very limited you may find that you need to stay in a circle throughout the session. The centre of the circle can then act as the platform for the story and people can come in and out as they please.

Participation

Depending on the aims of your particular work or project, it can help to tell adults from the outset that nothing is compulsory. If you find people abstaining before you've even explained the game or activity, encourage them to make this decision once they know what the exercise is, rather than before. Often those who do choose to opt out can still have a valuable experience from the sidelines and eventually feel more inclined to join in as they watch everyone else enjoying themselves.

There are many ways of allowing more shy group members to remain an important part of the story-making process. You could invite people to share their ideas by creating the sounds for the story using instruments and voice if they don't want to play a role. This is an important job but can be done discreetly if necessary. For those who are particularly resistant asking for their comments on the action can help to include them in the story-making session, although you will need to consider how having this observer might impact on the rest of the group.

When working with any age group, play is always the best place to start. Adult groups can often be sceptical when silly games are initiated, yet before long barriers drop and playfulness develops. Once play feels natural and comfortable then, just as it did in childhood, the stories will come.

CASE STUDY

In one care home, while working with a small group of elderly ladies with dementia, we were confronted with a participant who was extremely confused and anxious. While a member of staff tried to comfort her, a multi-coloured sensory ball was introduced to the group which instantly drew everyone's attention. As it was passed around, the lady started to quieten and appeared drawn in by the unusual object. When the ball was eventually passed to her, she beamed with delight, tossing the ball up into the air before passing it on. A connection between everyone in the room then developed and from this simple game a story was created.

The non-verbal, playful activity appeared to break the cycle of her anxiety and gave her a much-needed creative distraction. She then participated fully in the session and was able to work through some of her anxiety non-directly through the story-making process.

Observation

As a facilitator working with adults, try to maintain the belief that the barriers to playfulness will come down with time. Have faith in your abilities if the laughter dies away or the energy drops. The moments where people appear closed off might be the moments when they are most engaged, so try not to let it shake your confidence. You may find that there are times when people close their eyes or move away from the group, but they could be experiencing something internally which is not noticeable to the outside world.

Using a combination of intuition and good observation skills should allow you to assess how the session is going. Every gesture, word, glance and movement is a form of communication which can help you to understand your group's needs at any given moment.

Staying In Control

One of the most common worries for anyone introducing drama in the classroom or group setting is the fear of losing control; of the lack of discipline that could occur. A group engaged in drama activities can often appear chaotic. However, for the drama to work, rules and structure must be in place so the group can play effectively and successfully.

People working regularly within an SEN classroom or group setting will be used to managing unexpected situations and behaviour, even so, introducing drama into an ordered daily routine can be daunting. Although there is no substitute for preparation and planning, the following tips can help when it comes to managing a group and channelling the creativity of even the most highly energised participants.

CODE OF CONDUCT

When setting up a new project or regular group, ensure that all participants are aware of the group's 'Code of Conduct'. This is especially important when working with groups who have challenging behaviour.

As well as including rules, a Code of Conduct should outline the consequences should the rules be broken and group members could even be asked to sign the Code of Conduct as a form of contract before being allowed to participate.

Some groups might be able to develop the Code of Conduct for themselves. Starting with a basic list, they can then decide what is important for them. For example, one group might want to ban offensive language while for another, freedom of speech could be more important. One group might want to have a time-out chair for anyone who repeatedly behaves badly, while another might want to develop a system that puts the person on probation (this could eventually lead to their exclusion from the group should the behaviour continue).

This Code of Conduct could be reinforced through drama, with the group demonstrating a freeze-frame or tableau of unacceptable behaviour that could be photographed and displayed alongside the rules.

Allowing the group to have input into the rules and setting them out clearly in advance can often help with any challenging behaviours should they arise (although if an unexpected situation does occur, it can be the perfect opportunity to revise the Code of Conduct with the group).

ACCEPT, ACCEPT, ACCEPT

When working with a group, many different opinions and ideas can arise simultaneously. While it might not be possible to use or include all of the ideas, it is important that they are at least heard and acknowledged. Strategies can include writing down the person's name and their suggestion (and making sure they see you do so) or asking them to tell their ideas to a support worker. Breaking into smaller groups and asking these groups to share ideas with each other (or even just asking them to share their thoughts with the person beside them) can also satisfy the need to be heard and valued.

Very often group members will 'play up' if they feel ignored or undervalued, while others will deliberately try to test the boundaries put in place. Accepting their input, no matter how small or apparently inappropriate, can help to engage them more fully.

> ## CASE STUDY
>
> When working on 'The Last Drummer' project, a group of boys developed a scene that included a lot of swearing. Rather than tell them off, which they expected, we accepted their swearing scene but asked them whether their tribe would use recognised swear words, or have words unique to the village. The boys then reworked their scene and produced a brand new language, including imaginary swear words!

Learning to accept, transform and enhance ideas is a skill that professional improvisers develop with time and practise, in order to do so without the need to control, negate or fundamentally change the original idea.

MANAGING ENERGY

For aggressive or highly energetic participants who need extra management, use exercises that are designed to focus and calm a group down (or adjust games that require 'running around' to moving in slow motion). The following activities are just some examples of exercises that can help to manage energy.

> ### Activity: Movement Circle
>
> Put on some calming music and get the group sitting in a circle. Slowly start to move your arms, asking the group to copy you. Encourage participation by passing the lead on to others in the circle. This activity is ideal for creating focus and finishing a session.

> ### Activity: Go If
>
> Have the group sit on chairs in a circle with one person standing in the middle. The person in the middle says 'Go if ...' followed by a statement that is true about themselves. For example, 'Go if you have blonde hair'. Anyone with blonde hair who is sitting in the circle must then move to another chair. The person in the middle must try to sit on a chair. The person left standing in the centre starts the next round with a new suggestion.
>
> This game promotes listening skills while still allowing bursts of energy.

Activity: Slow-Motion Sword Fight

Invite the group to line up in front of you. In-role as the Master Sword Fighter demonstrate the following actions in slow motion (including exaggerated facial expressions). Explain that for every action you perform, there is a reaction they must perform.

★ Bend down and sweep your imaginary sword low to the ground.
   The group must jump high into the air.

★ Stretch up high and swing your imaginary sword above their heads.
   The group must duck down.

★ Jab to the right.
   The group move to the left.

★ Jab to the left.
   The group move to the right.

Practise a few times before stating that anyone who moves too quickly will be out. This activity is great fun, expels a lot of energy and promotes listening and observation skills.

For any exercise, set up chairs or mats for the group to return to should the exercise start to deteriorate and guide them in some group breathing. It's amazing how quickly three slow breaths in and out can calm and focus a group.

Keeping your voice calm will also have a big impact on the group. If the group is becoming unruly, bring one person at a time back to the chairs or mats, praising them for remaining calm.

Giving clear instructions as to what is going to happen is also important. For example, tell the group that you are going to ask them to stay frozen until you tap individuals on the shoulder. This will then be the cue for them to start their activity. Let them know in advance what the signal to 're-freeze' will be, such as clapping hands or tapping them on the shoulder again. Never be afraid to stop and start an exercise or drop role mid-activity in order to incorporate ideas or keep the group on track.

CASE STUDY

When working on 'The Sleeping Boy' project, a swamp was established through a soundscape activity which the group practised a few times. When they came to 'do it for real', the exercise was suddenly interrupted by a boy energetically running around the room pretending to be a Vampire Bat. Instead of seeing this as a disruption, we asked him to re-do his action and movement more slowly, incorporating it gradually into the original swamp soundscape. We then narrated this Vampire Bat character into the developing story and the group had a discussion on how this character's input affected the mood of the swamp. It took the story in a wonderfully unexpected direction.

STAGING A FIGHT SEQUENCE

Should you need to stage a fight as part of a performance, the movement sequence outlined in Handout 6 can help stage the scene safely and doesn't require a specialist fight choreographer. It is important to remind the group that *at no time do the actors make physical contact.*

CASE STUDY

I once staged a fight sequence for a production of 'Romeo & Juliet' with a group which included some wheelchair-users. On this occasion I worked with them to ascertain what movements they were comfortable with and we ended up with Mercutio calling out to his friend Romeo as he slowly climbed through an obstacle course of upturned wheelchairs.

Staging A Safe Fight Sequence

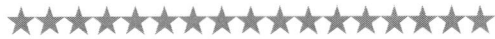

★★★★★★★★★★★★★★★★★★

1 Place two 'actors' on opposite sides of the room.

2 Ask them to develop three moves that can be repeated in sequence.

3 Each actor then performs their sequence, first one after the other and then simultaneously. Encourage them to make their moves big and in slow motion. Explain that this is 'stage fighting' so if they move too fast, the audience will not be able to see what's going on.

4 Once they have practised this a couple of times, ask them to move in a large circle around the edge of the room, slowly repeating their fight sequence as they move. (If possible, ask them to maintain eye contact with each other.) They could also move slowly towards each other, freezing before they finally meet.

5 Music could then be added to underscore the scene and the rest of the group might like to make suggestions or provide accompaniment using percussion instruments.

POWER STRUGGLES

A power struggle between participants can often take the form of 'He copied me'. One way of nipping this in the bud is to let the group know that if two or more people come up with the same idea then it must be an important one. (If there is a genuine issue of deliberate and consistent copying that is distressing for one person, you will need to address this separately.)

If a power struggle arises between natural leaders in a group, suggest that this role is shared or incorporate it into the story, for instance developing a ritual that has one leader 'pass on the baton' to another. If the rift continues, this lack of unity could become the focus for characters in the story.

Unfortunately, another power struggle that can occur is between a visiting practitioner and a group's regular teacher or within an organisation where someone is trying to introduce drama and play into the daily routine and having to convince others of its benefits.

Some teachers may interrupt a workshop in order to tell off a pupil who they feel is misbehaving. The child may be doing exactly what you have asked and this interruption and reprimand may lead to confusion as well as undermining you.

You may find that a group's regular leader interrupts or contradicts you. While accepting their need to be heard as much as possible, this can stifle the group's creativity as they feel a divided loyalty towards their regular teacher and the work you are asking them to do. You may occasionally find someone 'showing-off' to participants, which can also hinder the group's creative play. This showing-off is very different from having someone demonstrate an activity in order to inspire the group – perhaps the best way to distinguish between the two is to observe how much ego is involved.

It is difficult to manage these kinds of power struggles on-the-spot and it is unwise to undermine the regular teacher's authority in front of their class. This is why pre-workshop preparation and discussion is always wise (see 'Support Staff' above).

FINAL THOUGHTS

When introducing any new game, have a practice run. Sometimes groups will become unruly if they are not succeeding quickly enough or lack the concentration for a particular activity and feel out of their depth. Therefore, gradually build up exercises (see 'Breaking Down The Drama Game', p. 55), tell the group that you are going to have a practice run and inform them that this activity is very advanced, giving constant praise for even the smallest success.

Don't feel that it is solely your responsibility to discipline a group. As a visiting practitioner working with an established group, the regular support staff and teachers should be on hand to manage the group's behaviour. Again, set this out in advance.

You may find that your group behaves wonderfully well when their teacher is in the room but once left alone with you, their focus deteriorates and they misbehave. The sessions then become more of an exercise in crowd control than creative play. Discipline should not be left to one person; management strategies need to be established between you and the regular staff prior to any project or workshop.

Your energy and commitment is also vitally important. If you don't care about the workshop or story being created, why should they? Often groups with a lot of energy (even negative energy) are easier to work with as you can harness this energy and focus it into the developing drama. In contrast, groups with little motivation can be hard work, as the energy needed to motivate them can very easily wear you out.

No matter what level or type of energy the group has, positive reinforcement is vital. Anyone (teenagers and adults in particular) can feel very self-conscious when participating in drama for the first time. Rather than pushing them to join in fully from the beginning, accept their boundaries and praise any participation no matter how small. Some people may not want to join in; simply attending the group can be enough. You may find that eventually, in their own time, they join in the activities.

CASE STUDY

In one adult group there was a member with learning difficulties who refused to join in. He wanted to be there, but while the group was engaged he would sit at the side of the room. During the sessions I would often ask him quietly what he thought of the game being played or the drama being developed. When he did finally come and sit with us in the circle I commented positively saying how fantastic it was that he was with us. Eventually he started to participate in those activities he was comfortable with.

Although positive reinforcement is important, so is the need to be firm when inappropriate behaviour emerges. On one occasion, a girl in a regular group would have a tantrum if her idea was not heard first every time. It was made very clear that tantrums were not acceptable in the group and if she persisted we would ignore her. (This strategy was established in conjunction with her parents.) Another child would also have the occasional tantrum. However, when he did it was not ignored, as this behaviour was known to be the signal for something quite serious. Ultimately, trust your instincts. Managing any group is a creative process and what works for one person doesn't necessarily work for another.

Developing Your Own Storytelling Style

THE NATURAL STORYTELLER

Even if you have never told a story before in your life, you are still a storyteller. Telling stories is something we all do on a daily basis, often without thinking about it. People are naturally sociable and much of our social energy is taken up with storytelling. When you describe an event in your day to a friend or colleague, you are telling a story. How you tell this story will depend on your listener's response and your personal style of communication. However you choose to tell these stories is the right way for you; there is no 'perfect storyteller' or 'right' way to tell a story. Stories only truly exist as they are told; as a story is formed it can never be repeated in the same way again. Therefore, the way stories are devised and told is *right in that moment*.

Fundamentally, being a storyteller is about being *present* and being yourself. Whichever style of storytelling comes naturally to you will be engaging to those with whom you are working and will consequently generate a natural and truthful response from them, as long as *you* are engaged and present. Therefore, providing a 'how to' guide to storytelling is not meaningful or indeed, possible. Instead, the aim of this book is to help you develop your own storytelling style by offering you a series of concepts to consider, as a way of strengthening your own natural style. The intention is that these ideas will enhance your confidence as a storyteller and help you to develop your effectiveness, as opposed to creating a storytelling style from scratch. Begin with what you already have and then, if you find it helpful, consider the following.

USE OF VOICE & BODY

The way that you use your voice and body when leading the session will have a direct impact on the experience of the participants. That is not to say that voice is an imperative element of storytelling – it is entirely possible to create a story without using words at all. However, the majority of drama and story sessions will involve verbal communication and it is therefore worth considering your own approach. The way that you speak to the group should be completely natural to you but should also contain enough variety, contrast and energy to engage the listeners. Explore altering the rhythm and pace of your voice depending on what is happening in the story. Hushed whispers when approaching a cave or having a big, booming voice to represent a giant will all help enhance the excitement and adventure. Keep in mind the group you are working with when considering your pace and volume. Speaking too fast might lose people but speaking too slowly can appear patronising, while being too loud could upset those who are sensitive to sound.

Using gesture to emphasise your words will add a strong visual element and may make the story more accessible to those whose communication style is non-verbal. Also consider your posture and body language; leaning forward in your chair indicates that you are inviting the group to join you and engage with what you are saying. It is also great fun to be physical when telling stories and as the leader you can model this for the group. The characters in the story are likely to feel more real and engaging if embodied and enacted physically. Equally, moments of stillness will offer contrast and variation to the action where necessary.

FROM WITHIN

For hundreds of years traditional stories have been recounted orally and it is in the telling of them 'from within' that entrances the listener. Telling a story often is more effective and powerful when done impulsively and without a script. It is this spontaneous telling that creates the magic and life of a story in the moment that it is told. This method also allows you to make good eye-contact with your group, bringing the story to life through your facial expressions and body.

This doesn't mean that you have to learn a story by heart and recite it; it can be possible to recount a story in a matter of minutes if you think about it in the right way. As an exercise, read the story of 'The Return of the Flowers' (Handout 24) and as you are reading it, *picture* the story in your head. Then read it once more, fixing these pictures in your mind. Now run through the images with your eyes closed, without looking at the words of the story. Try not to think about the actual words that were written, but just see the story in the pictures you imagined. Now, using these pictures as a guide, try retelling the story out loud. Don't think about *remembering* the words of the story – just tell it as you see it in your head. It may come out quite differently from its original form, but that is what happens in oral storytelling; no story is ever told the same way twice. If you have children then you can always practice your storytelling on them and see how they respond (even getting them to add their own ideas).

ASK QUESTIONS

In order to facilitate the group's ownership of the story-making process, invite them to share their thoughts and ideas about the story by asking questions. *How* you phrase these questions is important to consider, so have a look at the following examples. When asking about the character of a dragon, you might ask:

"So, the dragon lives in this forest, does he? And is he a friendly dragon?"

In this example you can see that the facilitator is asking very leading questions, which only require 'yes' or 'no' answers. Simply by using the words 'forest' and 'friendly', the group are being limited in their choice and input, as the ideas are already formed by the questions. Instead, the question could be posed as follows:

"So, where does this dragon live?"

One person might say 'In a forest', whilst another might say 'In the sky'. You could then respond with:

"It sounds as if this dragon lives in a forest in the sky. Is that right? OK, let"s travel up to the sky and see what this 'sky forest' looks like."

And then:

"So what kind of dragon is he? Everyone call out your ideas!"

As the group call their ideas, simply echo what they say to emphasise that you have taken each response on board:

Participant 1:   *'Big!'*

Facilitator: *'OK, a big dragon, anything else?'*

Participant 2:   *'Smelly!'*

Facilitator: *'Oh, I see, a smelly dragon! What else?'*

Participant 3:   *'I think he's angry.'*

Facilitator: *'OK, so he's a big, smelly, angry dragon. Why don't we find out what he looks and sounds like?'*

Now you could get the group to make the shape of the dragon with their bodies, adding sounds to show his anger. (To avoid losing control in this kind of exercise, have the group sit as an audience and each person come up one at a time, to add themselves into the image. This also allows them to look and assess where they want to place themselves to form the dragon.) Whenever the dragon appears in the story (perhaps indicated by a sound cue), the group can reform into this shape as quickly as possible and make the dragon sounds. This then becomes a game within the story-making process.

When working with groups with more complex disabilities the group may find responding to questions, offering ideas or making choices more challenging. On these occasions you may need to lead the story a little more, while still giving the group choice. For example, when asking a group *'Who lives in this forest?'* you could show a number of puppets asking the group to indicate which character they think might live there.

Of course, it is not always possible to take on board and incorporate every idea, and part of this work is always going to be about compromise and managing fairness. If you find that you're struggling to maintain fairness when using ideas, then direct your questions at a specific person: 'So Ruby, where do you think this dragon might live?' If that person struggles to come up with an idea then other people can help her out and you can let her decide which idea to choose. As the group get to know you and each other, you will find that ideas flow more easily and you will become increasingly confident at managing this process effectively.

NARRATE WHAT YOU SEE

As the facilitator or story-leader, it is your job to listen and respond to what is going on in the room and this requires keen observational skills. Once the story-making process has begun and the group are engaged in the activities, you will find that the story starts to tell itself if you *narrate what you see*. To practise this, try the following activity.

Activity: Narrate What You See

1 In this exercise each person is invited to find a space in the room to 'build their home' in an imaginary village (this could be done with or without props and materials).

2 As the activity begins, narrate your observations about what is happening, for example:
'As each villager began building their home, everyone set about their tasks with care and attention.'

3 Ask the villagers what tools they are using to build their home and incorporate this into the story.
'One villager used a hammer, another stones and bricks and yet another used sand and water. Their tools made extraordinary noises that echoed throughout the night.'

---

4 Encourage each villager to explore the sounds and rhythms of their different tools. This could be through voice, use of the body or with musical instruments. In this way your narration has not only observed the action, but helped to guide the group.

5 Should any villager be reluctant to participate or have problems with their construction, this can also be incorporated into the narration. For example: 'But there was one villager who, despite putting in enormous effort, could not get his house to stay standing. Each time he put something up, it came tumbling down – BANG, CRASH! He began to feel frustrated and looked to see how the others were getting along. Another villager caught the man's eye and realised that he seemed to need some help...'

In this way, through narration, you will be able to start bringing the group's focus back together again, as they are given an opportunity to help somebody and attempt to solve the problem. From here the story might develop so that however hard they try, the villagers can't get this house to stay standing. Perhaps an old, wise lady then warns them that this spot was the site of a witch's curse, many years ago. The villagers might then decide that it is their job to find a way to break this curse so that the man in the village can build his house successfully!

Reluctant Participants

Part of narrating what you see is about drawing in those group members who are less confident about participating. In 'The Sleeping Boy' Workshop (p. 107), it was because of one boy's *actual* tiredness that this element of the story developed. It can be exciting and surprising for someone who does not feel part of the story to suddenly realise that a movement, action or sound they have made has been noticed by you and incorporated into the narrative. Of course, it is important to respect someone's choice not to participate if that is something you have agreed, but quite often such a person will be drawn into the story-making, almost without realising it. Be aware that if a person you are trying to draw into the narrative continues to display a negative response then it is likely to be too much too soon.

Redirecting The Story

One of the difficulties with narrating what you see is that the story may end up going in a direction that seems strange or difficult. Someone might have an idea, or do something, that you feel is 'not right' for the story, so try and assess why you are having this response. Is it because you are prioritising your own ideas over those of the participants, or is it in the best interests of the group and story? One reason to change the direction of the story is if you feel it is becoming consistently violent. For example, you may be working with a group of boys who keep wanting to stage fights. Battles in stories are fine to a certain extent (if you facilitate this safely), but become meaningless if they are the *only* direction the story goes in when there is a conflict.

Confidence

Narrating what you see must therefore be done with good awareness and careful judgement. This approach to storytelling is very person-centred and requires confidence regarding spontaneity on the part of the facilitator. It may be that you only narrate what you see once or twice during a session, while sticking closely to the session plan for the rest of the time. This doesn't make the work any less worthy; the crucial aspect of working in this way is to only do what feels natural and comfortable. If you try to facilitate in a way that makes you anxious, then it is likely to have a negative impact on the group dynamics anyway.

Narrating what you see may be as simple as verbalising small and intimate moments, which might otherwise go unnoticed: the sound of a voice, the shake of a scarf or a facial expression. By developing your storytelling style to incorporate keen observation and awareness of the group's behaviour, you may find that the smallest and apparently most insignificant moment becomes the central aspect of a story.

USE OF PROPS & COSTUMES

With any group, but especially when working with people who have learning or communication needs, offering a multi-sensory approach to drama and story-making is fundamental. The use of colour, shape, texture, sound, light and movement will enhance the group's experience and offer them a non-verbal way in to the process. For some people, an imagined story with no visual, auditory or kinaesthetic element can be too abstract and difficult to access. Stimulating the senses will offer the group a range of experiences, allowing them the opportunity to access the session according to their preferred learning style. Use of props can also add an element of mystery and excitement. In the 'Clue Bags' Workshop (p. 69), props are used as a series of clues to solve a mystery. Having props hidden away out of sight and then revealing them at particular moments can add to the adventure of the story and heighten levels of engagement.

Having your sensory storytelling kit to hand means that you can use the props as and when you need them. If you make your props accessible to support staff, they can also use them when providing one-to-one support, adding to the sensory experience. It can help if the props used are relevant to the theme of the story, for example if support staff use a spider puppet with someone when a spider has never appeared in the story, then the use of the prop becomes distracting and detrimental.

You may find that the use of props can support you in the development of your storytelling style. Props can be a great source of comfort to a story-leader as they offer something tangible to work with and can somehow make you feel less 'alone'. Try to think through in advance the props you might use in a session and how they could be used to guide and aid the story. You might also need to locate extra props as a story progresses and develops from week to week. If a gold crown becomes an important feature of a story then it may help to bring one in the following week. Of course, you will also have ideas about how to use a prop to enhance the story *in the moment*. Props can also help you out of challenging situations if you feel that the story is 'stuck': a rolled-up cloth in the corner of a room might suddenly become a magic carpet or the discovery of a fossil on the ground might provide a clue on the journey.

Using costumes depends entirely on the size of the group and the materials available to you. On the whole it is probably best to avoid using full costumes unless working with a really small group (two to four people). However, bits of costume such as hats, scarves and cloaks can be great. Pieces of fabric are the most adaptable props as they can also double as costumes. Try to collect material in a range of colours and textures, which can be used as cloaks or gowns, as well as being used to create environments.

You could also use the fabric for your own costume, aiding you if working in-role. If you have the confidence to assume a role from time to time, this can be a hugely effective aspect of your storytelling style. Using a piece of costume when in-role will make a clear distinction between when you are the story-leader, and when you are in character.

CASE STUDY

On one occasion during 'The Sleeping Boy' project I turned my back to the group and placed a black piece of material over my head and shoulders, changing my facial expression and posture, to become an evil witch. The children were excited by the sudden presence of this witch and were able to talk and respond to her as though she was real. Then, when necessary, I simply turned my back, took off the 'cloak' and became myself again, asking the children to tell me all about what they had just seen. Making this visual distinction allowed the children to believe in the character of the witch, while still knowing clearly that I was 'myself' when I was not wearing the witch's costume.

LEARN FROM OTHERS

Many different factors will have an impact on your storytelling style, but it's best not to worry about every detail as this can make you self-conscious. After all, your storytelling style should be about facilitating the process in a way that you are comfortable with and which you feel best engages your group. Your particular style will never appeal to everyone. You may find that some groups respond more positively to you than others, or that your style needs to be adapted slightly depending on who you are working with.

Above all, try to observe other facilitators, practitioners and teachers leading sessions, as you can learn much from how other people work.

Breaking Down the Drama Game

ADAPTING DRAMA GAMES

Many people feel that groups which include people with additional needs should have 'special' drama games, as they may see traditional games as unsuitable. However, if you understand the components of an activity and know what it aims to achieve, any drama game can be adapted for any group or individual.

When working with new groups you will need to do an assessment of needs – are they boisterous and in need of focus or reserved and in need of waking up? With groups who have different levels of needs you will also have to assess comprehension levels to some extent, and take into account practical considerations such as accessibility for wheelchair-users.

In time you will find that you are able to adapt a handful of favourite games for any eventuality, rather than trying to remember an infinite list of games. Instead of presenting a list of activities, this chapter will show how to break activities down into their component parts, giving you the tools to help you adjust traditional games to your group's needs, as well as invent new ones.

Game: Zip, Zap, Boing!

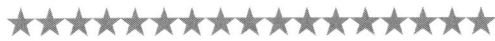

★★★★★★★★★★★★★★★★★★★★★

Rules of the Game

★ Ask the group to stand in a circle.

★ Choose someone to start.

★ The word 'Zip' is passed around the circle in one direction (a hand action can also accompany the passing of the word from one person to their neighbour).

★ Once the group is confident in passing 'Zip', introduce 'Zap' which can be sent anywhere across the circle.

★ Practise sending 'Zips' and 'Zaps'.

★ Once comfortable with 'Zips' and 'Zaps', introduce 'Boing!' which sends the 'Zip' or 'Zap' back to the person who sent it.

★ Remember though – you can't 'Boing!' a 'Boing!' – this will make sense when you try it!

Aims of the Game

Promoting eye contact, vocal development and group confidence.

Note

This game can take a number of practise sessions to get right. The group needs to work together with energy and commitment for it to succeed.

Adapting for Groups with Learning Difficulties

How could such a game be used with those who have trouble making eye-contact, speaking, hearing or even standing in a circle? The secret is to understand the *aims* and the *components* of the game and then to make adaptations to accommodate any physical or sensory needs.

One of the aims of 'Zip, Zap, Boing!' is to promote team work and one of the game's components is for the group to stand in a circle. If your group has severe learning, emotional or behavioural difficulties you could adapt the game as follows:

★ Draw a chalk circle on the floor.

★ Walk around the outside of the circle repeating the word 'Zip'.

★ Before you make a full rotation of the circle the group must form a circle.

★ When the last person is in place, everyone must say 'Zap'.

★ If you get around the circle first, you say 'Zap'.

★ As the group became more proficient at getting into a circle, increase the speed at which you walk.

★ You could also add appropriate rewards (e.g., stickers) for making it to the circle in time.

It could be argued that this creates a completely different game, but you should look at it as a building block. Not only does it stay true to the aims of 'Zip, Zap, Boing!' (groupwork, eye-contact, listening and speaking skills) but it is also helping the group to develop to a point where they might be able to start playing a version of the original game.

Another adaptation for a group of teenagers who may be hard to motivate is to replace the words 'Zip', 'Zap' and 'Boing!' with greetings suggested by the group. For instance, they might choose to pass 'Alright' around the circle, 'Wotcha' across the circle and replace 'Boing!' with 'Backatcha!'

CASE STUDY: Adaptation for Complex Disabilities

On one occasion this game was adapted to include a boy with complex disabilities. He liked to hold a red block and would get distressed if he couldn't see it in the classroom. He rarely engaged with the rest of the class, so to encourage him to participate in more groupwork, a simplified game of 'Zip, Zap, Boing!' was created.

- Before introducing the boy to the group, a support worker spent time with him in individual play, saying 'Zip' when the block was taken away from him and 'Boing!' when it was passed back.

- The rest of the group then sat in a circle and passed his red block around saying 'Zip' as they did so.

- He sat with his support worker watching his block go around the circle and when it finally reached him the entire group said 'Boing!'.

- To increase the drama, the direction of the red block would suddenly change just as it was about to reach him and slowly, as the rest of the group increased their skill, the idea of 'Zap' was introduced by having individuals say 'Zip' if they passed the red block to the person next to them, or 'Zap' if they passed it across the circle.

This activity could be turned into a group story that could be narrated while playing the game. For example, 'There was once a red block [the group bang blocks together or clap their hands] who had loads of energy. He would Zip around the room [the group say 'Zip'] looking for his very special friend…'

In this way, with the original game as inspiration and by staying true to its aims, not only is there a means of encouraging a hard-to-engage pupil into groupwork, but by 'narrating what you see' there is also the potential for creating a story.

Adaptation for Sensory Impairment

'Zip, Zap, Boing!' can also be adapted for groups with hearing and sight impairments by including an element of touch. The group could all sit on chairs and pass a 'Zip' around the circle by tapping the knee of the person next to them or passing around a soft ball. A 'Zap' could then involve throwing the soft ball across the circle, calling or signing the person's name as you do so. Wherever possible, try to include the group in the process of adapting the game by allowing them to problem solve and work it out together. If in doubt about whether anything will work, try a demonstration or practice session first.

BREAKING DOWN A GAME

Ask yourself:

1 What are the *Aims* of the game? For example, 'Zip, Zap, Boing!' is all about focus, working together, eye-contact, listening and speaking with confidence. Therefore any adaptation of the game should still promote some of these aims.

2 What are the *Components* of the game? For example, what step-by-step instructions do the group need in order for them to succeed at playing the game?

3 What *Sensory* (visual, hearing or mobility) adaptations need to be made in order to make the game accessible?

SAMPLE 'BROKEN-DOWN' GAMES

The following games have been categorised according to their main aim, although there are obvious crossovers. For example, in addition to building trust, 'Camera Blink' also requires a great deal of focus while 'Animal Chase Sounds' not only energises but also promotes groupwork.

As well as showing how these games can be adapted, you can use the format in the handouts (8–11) below when adapting your own activities.

Game: Camera Blink

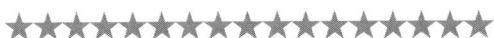

★★★★★★★★★★★★★★★★★★★★

AIMS

★ To develop **trust** between group members.

★ To discover a new way of looking at familiar things.

HOW TO PLAY

★ Form pairs and ask one person to close their eyes. This person is the 'camera'.

★ The 'camera' is then led gently around the room by the other person.

★ From time to time, the person leading can stop and gently squeeze the hand of the 'camera'. When this happens, the 'camera' quickly opens and closes their eyes taking a mental picture of the image in front of them.

★ Set up some interesting shots for the camera or get the 'leaders' to do so.

★ After a couple of minutes the pairs can swap roles.

★ Discuss afterwards how this felt and what was seen.

COMPONENTS

★ Working in pairs.

★ Holding hands.

★ Walking responsibly.

★ Opening and closing eyes.

SENSORY ADAPTATIONS

★ If your group cannot work responsibly in pairs, then set up the activity in front of the group with you guiding each 'camera' and have the rest of the group create an interesting scene (either using objects or their own bodies).

★ For those with a visual impairment, set up items for the 'camera' to touch or even smell.

This page may be photocopied for instructional use only. *The Stories Within* © Sheree Vickers & Rosie Emanuel 2011

Game: Count 21

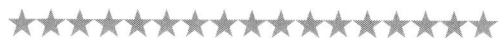

AIM

★ To develop **focus** between participants.

HOW TO PLAY

★ Standing in a circle, the group must count up to 21 with people calling out the numbers from 1 to 21, but without going around the circle.

★ If two people speak at the same time, they must start again at 1.

COMPONENTS

★ Standing in a circle.

★ Speaking, listening and working together.

SENSORY ADAPTATIONS

★ For groups with a short attention span reduce the number to 10 and remind them that it's not a race.

★ For those with hearing impairment, give each person a ball and invite them to throw their ball into the middle of the circle, one at a time. If two people throw their ball into the centre of the circle at the same time, they must start again. Keep trying until all the balls have been thrown.

Game: Animal Chase Sounds

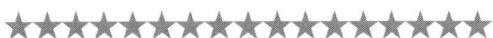

★★★★★★★★★★★★★★★★★★

AIMS

★ To help **energise** a group.

★ To promote speaking and listening skills.

HOW TO PLAY

★ Ask the group to stand in a circle.

★ Pass a 'meow' around the circle (possibly accompanied by a movement).

★ Once the group are comfortable passing this animal sound, introduce a 'woof'. So, as the cat sound is halfway around the circle, introduce the dog to chase the cat!

★ Slowly introduce more animals into the 'chase' circle.

★ For really advanced groups, have one animal going in one direction with another going the opposite way. Great fun when they cross over!

COMPONENTS

★ Standing in a circle.

★ Making animal sounds.

★ Staying focused.

★ Working as a team.

SENSORY ADAPTATIONS

★ Stuffed animals could be passed around the circle instead of making sounds.

★ For those with complex disabilities, sounds could be programmed into personal communication devices and then conducted like an orchestra. Alternatively the leader could walk around the circle saying 'meow' waiting for someone to say 'woof' which then sends the 'meow' in the opposite direction.

Game: Go If...

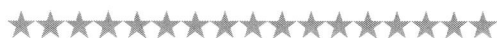

AIMS

★ To promote **interaction** within the group.

★ To learn more about each other.

★ To encourage confidence.

HOW TO PLAY

★ Have the group sit on chairs in a circle.

★ Standing in the centre of the group, say 'Go If ...' followed by something that applies to you. For example, 'Go if ... you are wearing black shoes' or 'Go if ... you like eating ice-cream.'

★ Everyone who agrees with the statement, or to whom it applies must move from their chair to another. Meanwhile you try and find yourself a spare chair.

★ The person who is left without a chair in the centre of the circle then starts a new 'Go If ...'

COMPONENTS

★ Sitting in a circle.

★ Listening and making connections between what's being said and your own situation.

★ Being able to move from one chair to another.

SENSORY ADAPTATIONS

★ If someone needs help to participate in the game then invite a support worker to be their partner for the duration of the game.

HANDOUT 11

★ In order to support those who might not be able to move quickly, tell everyone that they must move in slow motion (this also helps to keep people calm and focused).

★ Transform this into a mobile version of 'Snap' by giving out picture cards to each person. A pile of matching cards is then placed in the centre of the circle and the person in the middle holds up a chosen card. If anyone has the matching picture (or word) then they must move chairs.

★ If you have wheelchair-users in the group then mark out a place for each person on the floor using chalk or tape. (Those not in a wheelchair should be standing so that there are no obstructions to any of the positions in the circle). When people move, they must find a new marking on the floor, rather than a chair.

INCORPORATING GAMES INTO A STORY WORKSHOP

Often, drama games are used in isolation to warm-up, begin and end a session or as simple time fillers. Although it is fine to return to favourites in this way, drama games can also be a wonderful way of developing a story. For example, the 'McPuppet Locations' activity in 'AZ & McPuppets' is an adaptation of the traditional 'Compass Game' where North, South, East and West are replaced with different areas of the restaurant.

> ### Activity: The Compass Game
>
> The points of the compass (North, South, East and West) are written down and then stuck on the walls of the classroom. The leader calls out one of the 'points' and the group must assemble under that particular mark. An activity can be attached to each compass point. For example, when 'North' is called the group not only assembles at the North point, but must hop up and down/shake their heads/turn in a circle.

In the 'Romeo & Juliet' Workshop (p. 185), the masked ball includes the 'Mirror Game' as a way of having the Capulets challenge any possible Montagues at the party. The same game is also used by the mermaids as a challenge in the 'Lake' activity in 'The Falling Star' workshop (p. 193).

> ### Activity: The Mirror Game
>
> Facing each other in pairs, one person starts slowly moving. Simultaneously, the other person must then copy these movements as accurately as possible, as though looking in a mirror.

It is also important to keep in mind the pace of different activities. For instance, try to follow an energetic activity with a game that requires some stillness (e.g., 'Tunnel of Spiders' in 'The Sleeping Boy' Workshop (p. 107). This helps to keep focus and provides a different dynamic to the workshop and story being developed.

INAPPROPRIATE GAMES

Although any game can be adapted and used with any group, it is important to think carefully about the appropriateness of a particular game, bearing in mind who you're working with. For example, 'Falling Circle' is a trust game that involves a ring of people surrounding someone who is instructed to fall in any direction, expecting to be caught by the rest of the group. It is unwise to use this game with a group you don't know well or a group who are new to each other. Inappropriate games are those that counteract their aims. When used with a group who are not ready, 'Falling Circle' can rapidly deteriorate into chaos, removing any trust that might have already existed within the group.

If you are in any doubt, go back to the aims of the game and assess whether or not you think your group are ready to face the challenges that the particular game might offer.

PART II

Drama & Story Structures

INTRODUCTION

Each of the following drama and story structures were developed with a group that included participants with a wide range of needs. The workshops were sufficiently pre-planned to allow each of the groups the opportunity to play and have their own input into the developing story. None of these plans should be seen as set in stone. Instead, treat them either as a springboard or as a safety net to retreat to should the workshop become stale or the group need extra guidance.

For example, when developing the story of 'The Disappearing Monkeys' the character of Whale Shark appeared. He was large and hungry and drank not only the water, but also any creature that ventured close to the river's edge. If you are using this story structure as a springboard, the group could decide that the character of Whale Shark might be something (or someone) different, which will lead the other characters to travel to another location or environment. Alternatively, the character might not appear in your story at all, as the water and animals could be disappearing due to the effects of global warming!

In the story of 'The Sleeping Boy' the group developed a village with a problem. A wicked Enchantress cursed it so a young boy would sleep for a hundred years. In your own storytelling it could transpire that someone is sleeping for a reason that has nothing to do with an Enchantress casting a spell. In fact, the story might not even be about sleeping, but about some other problem the villagers have. For example, the village cook might need a special ingredient for a long-lost recipe, or the camels have escaped and the quest could be to find them.

It is also possible to mix and match activities from different workshops. For example, the 'Looking at Pictures' opening activity in 'The Last Drummer' could provide the visual stimulus for a story based on the theme of aggressive behaviour. This could then be followed by the 'Romeo & Juliet' structure, which could lead into a puppet-making workshop (such as those used in 'AZ & The McPuppets'), allowing the group to explore behaviour through the safety of character puppets.

Although these workshops have been used and developed in group settings, it is important to emphasise that they can also be adapted for use at home, or in any one-to-one situation.

It is recommended therefore, that you use the following plans as part of your storytelling 'toolkit' and have fun playing – often the most satisfying workshops can occur when the plan is either abandoned or adapted on the spot to accommodate the ideas of the group. When this happens, both the joy of creating together and the stories important to the group will emerge.

A Mystery Drama in One Session
Clue Bags

ORIGINAL SETTING

The aim of the 'Clue Bags' workshop was to give groups of young people the chance to create an original murder mystery story in one 90-minute session. Some of the young people involved had recently been to see a 'Whodunit' play at the theatre and so the workshop was linked to this experience. It was hoped that the process would offer groups an opportunity to develop their storytelling skills, enhance their creativity, and further explore the themes of the play.

The group consisted of smaller groups of young people aged 12 to19 years. Everyone involved had moderate learning disabilities or emotional and behavioural difficulties and we were able to gather a certain amount of information from teachers beforehand regarding the specific needs of each group. This was crucial as it meant that we had some idea of what to expect and could plan accordingly. Despite having this background information, we needed to create a workshop that was flexible enough for us to adapt to the needs of individuals in the moment, as the information only provided a very general picture. The workshop needed to provide a structure that could be adapted according to the different ages; being playful and simple enough for younger participants, while still challenging some of the older groups.

We wanted to use a multisensory approach and felt that the most appealing element of the play was its intrigue as a murder mystery. The workshop developed into the idea of each group creating their own 'Whodunit' story using a series of props and costumes as clues. This framework meant that we could give more freedom to some participants whilst being more directive with groups with higher support needs.

The Clue Bags themselves proved to be a very successful starting point for every group and highlighted the importance of tactile objects when engaging the imaginations of groups with a variety of learning needs. The costume pieces also provided a useful visual aid when character-building, enabling participants to easily move in and out of role.

The feedback received after each workshop was very positive. Using the theme of murder mystery seemed to have universal appeal to the young people involved. You may find that the workshop theme links well with a theatre visit or piece of literature being studied. It will also work successfully as a stand-alone workshop for any group.

PREPARATION

This workshop requires good support and a level of confidence on the part of the facilitator. Do have faith in your group; you should find that once inhibitions have dropped the majority of participants will engage fully in the process, devising incredibly funny, gritty and often meaningful stories in a very short space of time.

Keep in mind that some members of your group might need reassurance that the story being created is only pretend. By enhancing playfulness and ensuring that support workers keep an eye on people's responses, you should be able to have fun with this theme without it causing any problems.

Props & Materials

★ Three opaque drawstring bags, e.g., small laundry bags, to act as the Clue Bags.

★ A label for each bag – either a sticker or paper luggage label (Handout 12).

★ A large key (the older and bigger the better, or you could make one).

★ An old-looking landscape map (a bit like a 'treasure' map) marked with a cross stating 'You Are Here', a wiggly line to follow and then another cross at the end of the line. (This map could be made to look old by soaking blank paper in a shallow bowl of tea. Feel free to add small details such as trees, a swamp, an old house or a bridge.)

★ Two pre-written secret notes (Handout 12).

★ Pens and paper.

★ Notes with 'GUILTY' written on them, enough for each person in the group.

★ A soft ball for the warm-up game.

★ Five simple pieces of costume suggesting a mixture of male and female characters, for example:

   – silly glasses

   – a male hat

   – a female hat

   – a scarf or tie

   – plastic goggles

★ Five props which will act as clues to the motives of the five suspects, for example:

   – a pearl necklace

   – an old family photo

   – a pack of cards

   – a newspaper

   – a pocket watch

Clue Bags: Labels & Notes

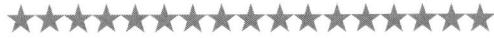

★★★★★★★★★★★★★★★★★★★★

WHERE?

WHO?

WHY?

Note 1

Murders happen when you least expect them ... trust no-one! Michael Jones aged 34 is dead! He was poisoned in a murder most horrid. You have one hour to discover who did it. The bags will help you. Good luck!

Note 2

Well done. You have found the scene of the crime but you still don't know 'whodunit'! Perhaps you need some more clues ...

Setting Up

The Clue Bags

★ Label each of the three bags with a sticker or luggage label:

  1 WHERE?

  2 WHO?

  3 WHY?

★ Place items inside each bag as follows:

  Clue Bag 1: WHERE?

  – The key

  – The map

  Clue Bag 2: WHO?

  – The five pieces of costume to create the suspects

  Clue Bag 3: WHY?

  – The five props to create the motives

★ Place the three Clue Bags somewhere at the side of the room where they are easily accessible to both you and the participants.

The Secret Notes

You will need to create two secret, worn-looking notes to be 'found' by you or a support worker at different moments in the storytelling process (see Handout 12).

Note 1 should be stuck on a wall or notice board, placed on the floor in a corner, or slotted into a door frame, anywhere it will not be spotted when participants enter.

Make sure that you give the group a specific cause of death for your victim (in this case poisoning) or you could end up with a workshop exploring ways to kill people! If you choose a different name or cause of death, remember to adjust your note accordingly.

Note 2 should be kept in someone's pocket or on a table with the rest of the props, to be brought out later in the proceedings.

THE STORY STRUCTURE

Introduce the concept of murder mystery to the group and begin creating a sense of intrigue and mystery by narrating something along the following lines, as dramatically as possible:

> *"Welcome everyone. Today you're going to need your wits about you. I've just heard that somewhere nearby a murder has taken place! Today your job is going to be to discover what happened and, of course, who did it! Every single person in this room is a suspect so remember to trust no-one..."*

Story-Building Activities

Now introduce the first of the drama activities 'I Didn't Do It' (see overleaf). This will help the group to relax and begin to assume roles.

Activity: Name Game – 'I Didn't Do It!'

This activity will help groups to begin exploring being in-role as a suspect and also adds a strong playful element at the start of the workshop. It will also help you to learn names if you don't know the group.

★ Use a soft ball that can be thrown or passed around the circle. As each person receives the ball they say 'I didn't do it, [James] did it!' and then pass the ball to the person they are 'accusing'.

★ As the game progresses, encourage everyone to become increasingly over-the-top in their statements, as if they are trying their best to convince everyone wholeheartedly that they 'Really, *really* didn't do it!'

★ Once the game is up and running you can start to playfully question certain people by saying to the group: 'Hmm, I'm not sure if I believe her, does anyone else? She sounds a bit suspicious to me!'

★ At the end of the game you could ask the group who they think did it and who sounded the most 'guilty'.

Note: There is a simplicity to this game that makes it accessible to everyone, even those who have more complex communication needs. If some members of your group are non-verbal or don't feel able to speak in front of others, invite them to prove their 'innocence' when they receive the ball through gesture or mime rather than words. This will also demonstrate to the group that people's gestures and facial expressions also provide clues in murder mysteries, as well as what they say.

CASE STUDY

You may find that people who are more confident with drama start to improvise and ad-lib new lines when they receive the ball. One particularly theatrical group member started exclaiming 'Hey, hang on a minute! You're accusing me? Well I can tell you absolutely, categorically, without a shadow of a doubt that I DID NOT DO IT!' If this happens then great, just ensure that everyone gets a chance with the ball and that you don't allow the more confident people to take over.

Activity: Wink Murder

It is not essential for everyone to be able to wink in order to play this game. As a group you could decide on a different signal for the chosen 'murderer' to use to 'kill' people in the circle. It needs to be a reasonably subtle signal such as a wink or blink, but could even be something like a big grin (therefore 'Grin Murder'!) or a hand gesture.

★ Once you choose your signal, go around the circle getting everyone to demonstrate it before you start the game, to ensure that it is something that everyone in the group can do comfortably, with support if necessary.

★ Explain that if they get winked/blinked/grinned at, then they can 'die' as dramatically as they like; you could ask a few people to demonstrate a dramatic death!

★ You will need a detective and a murderer; choose the detective first. If no-one volunteers, suggest that someone take on the role alongside a support worker.

★ Next choose a murderer. Ask the group to close their eyes while you tap someone on the shoulder (the detective should close their eyes too).Once the murderer is chosen, invite the detective into the centre of the circle. The murderer then begins to subtly 'murder' people using the agreed signal.

★ The detective must rotate slowly, looking around the circle, so that the murderer has a chance to deliver their signal when the detective's back is turned. Without this, the game can fail, as the murderer never gets a chance to give their signal without being immediately spotted by the detective.

★ The detective should be given three guesses as to who the murderer is.

★ Play the game a few times, as it may take a while for the group to get the hang of it if they have never played before.

Discovering the First Note

Once the group is comfortably playing 'Wink Murder', interrupt the proceedings by drawing the group's attention to the first note. Remember to add to the mystery by feigning ignorance and repeating any necessary information. You may say something along the following lines:

FACILITATOR: Um, sorry everyone… just hold on a minute. Is that someone's note on the [wall/door/floor]? Does it belong to anyone here?

PARTICIPANT 1: I bet you put it there Miss!

FACILITATOR: I've only just got here! How could I have put it there?

PARTICIPANT 2: It wasn't there before.

FACILITATOR: Do you think we should read it?

PARTICIPANT 3: Yeah, I'll get it! [He gets up]

FACILITATOR: OK, but don't read it yet. Just bring it over here. Do you want to read it? Stand here then and speak clearly so everyone can hear you. [Offer support as needed.]

PARTICIPANT 3: [Reading Note 1] 'Murders happen when you least expect them… Trust no-one! Michael Jones, aged 34, is dead! He has been poisoned in a murder most horrid! You have one hour to discover who did it. The bags will help you. Good luck!'

FACILITATOR: Michael Jones is dead! Does anyone know this Michael Jones? And poisoned! Wow, I wonder who would have done something like that! So what did it say? You have one hour to discover who did it using the bags to help you… What does that mean?

PARTICIPANT 4:   What bags?

PARTICIPANT 5:   Over there! *[Pointing to the 3 Clue Bags]*

FACILITATOR: Oh right, do you think that's what it means? Well, we'd better go and see. Would you like to go and see which bag we should start with? *[Go with them to the bags and ensure that they pick bag Number 1: WHERE?]*

Clue Bag 1 – WHERE?

★ Bring the first Clue Bag (containing the map and the key) into the centre of the circle. This Clue Bag will help the group to decipher *where* the murder has taken place.

★ Ask someone to put their hand inside the bag and pull one of the objects out (this always causes a lot of intrigue and laughter). Get someone else to pull out the second item.

★ Now use the map and key to discover where the murder took place.

The Map

★ First, ask the group what they think the clues might mean – take on board their ideas and eventually you should get to a point where someone says that *the map might lead to the location of the murder.*

★ Ask this person if they can be in charge of 'map-reading' and also ensure that the person who pulled out the key keeps it with them (if it's on a string then they could put it round their neck or wrist).

★ Break out of the circle and get everyone to line up behind the map-reader (as in 'follow-the-leader') to begin their journey into an imaginary world. The map-reader (with support if necessary) can use the wiggly line on the map to lead the group around the room, miming various movements to help denote each location. For example, the journey could involve crossing a range of environments such as wading through rivers, climbing mountains, crawling through forests, jumping over streams and squelching in mud. Alternatively the group might explore different rooms in an old house or a series of tunnels underneath the city.

★ As the journey progresses, ask the group to say what they can see and ask them to add sound effects where necessary.

★ Get the map-reader to shout out when they think they have reached the position marked by the map.

The Key

★ Once you've completed the initial journey, gather everyone around and draw their attention back to the key. Ask the group: 'What do you think this key might open?' Suggestions could include: 'A doorway/ trapdoor/ castle/ dungeon/ derelict house.'

★ Once you have a variety of ideas, make a decision about which one to go with, based on what you feel would work best for the group.

★ Using narration, get the group to help you create the imagined world for where the key will be used, for example: 'I think I can see the derelict house up there on the hill; let's approach it really quietly in case anyone is around. Can anyone see what it looks like yet? Oh, old and grey with ivy growing on the walls? Do you think we should go in?'

★ Now invite the person with the key to slowly unlock the imaginary door. The rest of the group could add sound effects and even create the shape of the doorway with their bodies for everyone to travel through.

★ Pretend to lock the door behind everyone and ask the group to describe what they can see and hear in this location. The group could even create a soundscape to enhance the atmosphere.

Discovering the Second Note

At this point you need to draw the attention to Note 2, which could be subtly dropped on the floor by you or a support worker and picked up by a member of the group. The exchange could go something like this:

FACILITATOR: *[Having dropped the note]* Sorry everyone, what's that on the floor?…

PARTICIPANT 1:   Another note!

FACILITATOR: Well you'd better have a look at it then. Can you read it out for us?

PARTICIPANT 2:   *[Reading Note 2]* 'Well done. You have found the scene of the crime but you still don't know whodunit! Perhaps you need some more clues…'

PARTICIPANT 3:   The clue bags! It's time for the next one.

FACILITATOR: OK, go and have a look and see which one you think will help us next. *[Offer support here if needed]*

PARTICIPANT 3:   Well, this one says number 2, so it must be this one. 'WHO?'

[The participant brings Clue Bag 2 to the group]

You will find that by this stage groups are much more willing to go along with the imaginary mystery of the story. At the beginning, some people may enjoy trying to break the illusion by saying things like '*You* put that note there' or 'I can't see any mountains, only the school hall!' You should find that even the most cynical group members will become swept up in the imaginary game by the time the second note is read out. If you do find that some refuse to go along with the concept then play along with this. You could draw them in by saying that their behaviour makes them appear very suspicious: 'Perhaps we should all be wary of [Simon]. Remember to trust no-one… and he seems to be especially keen to distract us all from finding out whodunit!'

Clue Bag 2 – WHO?

Clue Bag 2 contains the costume pieces that will help the group to create the possible suspects in the murder.

★ Once the second Clue Bag has been brought over, keep hold of it and ask the group what they think might be inside. Allow them to feel the bag to help them try and guess.

★ You now need to split into small groups of no more than five people. If you don't know the group well then ask a support worker to help, as they will have a better idea of who can work together. Try and get a good mix of abilities in each group, so that those with more confidence can help those who might need more support to voice their ideas.

★ Ask each group to find a space in the room and then take the Clue Bag round, letting each group pick out one item from the bag.

★ Tell each group that they need to choose one person to wear the piece of costume. This person is going to be in-role as a suspect, although you don't need to tell them this initially as this may put them off.

★ You should now have up to five people in the room wearing an item of costume. Narrate the following instruction to the groups:

"In your groups, it is now your job to create the suspects in this murder mystery. Each group will create a suspect profile using their piece of costume to help them. I want you to decide on the following: the name, the age and the profession of this suspect and, most importantly, their relationship to the victim. Remember that Michael was 34 years old when he was murdered, but that's all we really know about him."

It can be helpful to have the instructions printed on a worksheet for each group, with gaps for them to fill in the information. Use the template provided in Handout 13, or create your own.

★ When the groups are creating their suspect characters, try and steer them away from deciding on a specific motive at this point, as this is the next part of the story-making process, although you may want to ask them to 'hold that thought' for later.

★ Give the group about five minute to complete this task and make sure that everyone has finished before you move on.

Note: It is vital that as the facilitator, you move around each of the groups, keeping an eye on the ideas that come up. It's especially important that you keep track of their character's relationship to the victim, as it can get complicated if two groups claim to be Michael's mother! If this happens then you can either decide to nudge one group in a different direction or try and incorporate it into the next part of story (Clue Bag 3). For example, if you end up with Michael having two wives, then this could be a vital twist in the tale. Perhaps Michael didn't tell one wife that he was already married and this betrayal was her motivation to murder him!

Meet & Question the Suspects

★ Set up a line of chairs in a row as though facing an audience.

★ Invite each person who has chosen to wear the costume (and therefore play the suspect) to take a seat on one of the chairs. Get everyone else to sit facing them.

★ Explain to the suspects that they will need to think about their relationship with the victim and why they might have had reason to murder him.

★ If any of the suspects are reticent then explain that they don't have to say anything if they don't want to, or ask a support worker to play the 'voice' of the character by standing behind them, working as a team.

★ Ask each of the small groups to introduce their suspect, using the information from the previous activity (name, age, etc.).

★ As each suspect is introduced, it may be helpful to write their name and the other details on a piece of paper, placing it at their feet. This will act as a reminder of each character's name and will save you from remembering a lot of information.

Clue Bags Suspects

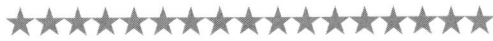

★★★★★★★★★★★★★★★★★★★★

★ **NAME**

_____

★ **RELATIONSHIP TO MICHAEL JONES**
   (e.g., family, friend, colleague, stranger)

_____

_____

★ **AGE**

_____

★ **PROFESSION/JOB**

_____

_____

_____

★ Once each character has been introduced by their group, take on the role of a detective by asking direct questions of suspects and inviting the audience to also ask questions. Keep this very simple, drawing out a few more details from each suspect.

As well as discovering any further information, this questioning will give the suspects a chance to get into character. If anyone playing a suspect is very quiet or shy then don't let this worry you. You can easily incorporate this into the story by playfully suggesting that perhaps their silence is their way of withholding evidence. Remember that as the facilitator you can pick up on particularly interesting comments or questions and guide the process to some extent. Your key role is to begin drawing out tensions between the suspects and the victim; there needs to be some evidence emerging at this point that will lead to a motive in the next part of the story.

★ Ask a support worker (in role as your 'assistant') to make a few notes about any evidence that comes up on each of the suspects. You may begin something like this:

FACILITATOR: *[In-role as a detective]* So here they are, our five suspects. And we know for a fact that one of you is the murderer! As suspects you all had a reason for wanting him dead, and we need to find out what these reasons (or motives) were. Only one of you did it... the other four are innocent!

Let's start with you [Suspect 1]. So you were Michael's [work colleague]. Who was in charge, you or him?

SUSPECT 1:   He was in charge – he was my boss. Very bossy.

FACILITATOR: Ah, so he liked bossing you around did he? And how did that make you feel?

SUSPECT 1:   Angry – he never let me get a word in!

Continue this dialogue until you have questioned every suspect. By now you should have a good sense of each character and know a little about why they had bad feelings towards the victim.

Clue Bag 3 – WHY?

Once each suspect has been questioned and you have a clear picture of each character's relationship to the victim, collect the final Clue Bag and tell the group that it is now time to find out *why* each of these characters might have wanted the victim dead – their motive. It might also be helpful to recap the information you have about each suspect so far to form a clear picture for everyone, using any notes that have been written down.

★ Tell the audience (all those not playing the role of a suspect) that they need to concentrate really hard now, as it will soon be up to them to make a decision on 'whodunit'!

★ Go to each suspect in turn and get them to reach inside the final Clue Bag and pull out an object.

★ It is now the job of the audience to speculate (through discussion) how each object provides a clue as to the motive of each suspect.

Following are some examples of how the story might evolve from here:

Suspect 1 'Mary Lynn'

One suspect, wearing a large straw hat, is the victim's wife – 'Mary Lynn'. We already know that their relationship has been rocky for the last few years and that Mary has been concerned as to why Michael often seems to stay late at work. We have also learned that the previous evening, Michael did not come home at all.

Motive Example 1, Clue: a pearl necklace
The group decided that Mary found the pearl necklace in her husband's coat pocket. Alongside the necklace was a love letter to Mary's sister. Mary then realised that her husband was having an affair with her sister and the betrayal was enough for her to want him dead!

Motive Example 2, Clue: a pack of cards

The group decided that Michael's absence from home was because he had a gambling addiction and had gambled away their life savings during long nights in the casino. One day Mary checked the accounts and realised what had happened. She is so angry that she lashes out and kills him!

Suspect 2 'Charlie'

This suspect, wearing some plastic goggles, is Michael's half-brother Charlie – a scientist. It has been established that Charlie and Michael have only recently found out about each other and that they have the same father. We also know that Charlie did not take the news well, as he found out that his father had a long, secret affair with Michael's mother and never told his wife.

Motive Example 1, Clue: a pocket watch

The group decided that the pocket watch was an old and extremely valuable family heirloom belonging to Charlie and Michael's father. A few days before Michael's death, Charlie had discovered that his father had decided to give the heirloom to Michael, rather than him. This news brought out all the anger and hatred towards Michael, to the point where Charlie may have wanted Michael dead.

Motive Example 2, Clue: a newspaper

The group decided that Charlie opened the newspaper one morning to discover that Michael had sold their controversial family story to the papers. However, he had only managed to sell the story by writing a whole heap of lies about Charlie and his mother, resulting in Charlie losing his job and his mother becoming a laughing stock. The deceit and outcome of Michael's actions was enough for Charlie to want him dead!

★ Once all the clues have been revealed and you have a motive for each suspect, it is your job to recap the evidence in a simple, clear and concise way.

★ Don't worry if you can't remember everything. The chances are that someone in the group will remember the details for you. Your role as storyteller when recounting each suspect's story is to make it sound as dramatic as possible. Murder mysteries tend to lean heavily towards melodrama, so feel free to use this approach when telling each suspect's tale.

Whodunit?

★ Once you have recounted each suspect's story, it is time to invite the group to make a decision about 'whodunit'.

★ Give them a few moments to think about this as you hand each group member a note with 'Guilty' written on it.

★ Invite each person to come up in turn and place their note at the feet of whichever suspect they think committed the murder.

★ Build up the tension as each vote is cast by commenting on who is currently looking most guilty.

★ When everyone has cast their vote, you will have solved the mystery as the suspect with the most votes is the murderer! Ask this character to stay where they are while the others de-role (by removing their costume) and receive a round of applause before joining the audience.

★ If two suspects end up with an equal number of votes, either combine their motives so it is possible that both committed the murder or, as the detective, you might need to cast a deciding vote.

★ Once the 'murderer' is left on their own, recount the story for the final time.

★ Ask the murderer if they have anything final that they want to say, then ask the person playing this character to take off their costume and welcome them back, by name, into the group with a round of applause.

At the end of the voting process you could summarise the story in the form of a case report. If you need time to work on this or don't feel confident enough to recount the story spontaneously then you can always do so after a break or in the next session. Alternatively it could springboard into some literacy work for the group.

THE MURDER OF MICHAEL JONES

Detective's report on the murder of Michael Jones.

It was discovered, after much questioning and forensic work, that Mary-Lynn, the deceived and tragic wife of the deceased, was indeed the murderer.

After many years in a rocky marriage, Mary was getting fed up spending long evenings on her own, while Michael 'worked late'. She had her suspicions, but was too frightened to question him. Then, one day he did not come home at all. She decided to take action and started searching through his belongings. And that was when she found a pearl necklace in the pocket of his coat! And not only that, but a love letter too! As she read the letter in horror she realised that the necklace was not just for any other woman but was in fact for her own sister! What a betrayal! She couldn't stand it. The deceit was too much to tolerate. The next day she went out to the chemist and bought the ingredients to create a poisonous mixture. She poured this into a bottle of wine and left it there for Michael to find when he came home that evening. The deed was done!

So ends this tragic tale.
Case Closed.

FURTHER DEVELOPMENT

Although this workshop was originally developed as a one-off for teenagers within mainstream or SEN settings, it could also be effectively used for groups of any age and delivered over a number of sessions. The following are examples of ideas for exploring or extending the work further.

★ Once the murderer has been discovered, take the individual or group on the return journey, using the key to release everyone from the location, having them retrace their steps using the map as a guide (over the rivers, or through the tunnels etc.).

★ The group might like to recreate what happened on the night of the murder. This could be done in the form of tableaux, getting small groups to develop the still images leading up to the poisoning and the aftermath.

★ Rather than casting individuals as each suspect, 'Role-on-the-Wall' can be used to develop the characters. Draw the outline of a person on a large piece of paper and get the group to speculate on the suspect's name, age and job, writing their ideas around the outside of the outline. Inside the shape write how the suspect might feel towards the victim and their relationship to him.

★ For those with more complex disabilities, this tactile workshop can be used to create stories in a smaller group or one-to-one setting. For example, a simple narrative could be developed by getting individuals to pull items (or pictures) out of a Clue Bag while you create a story that includes each of them in turn. For instance, 'Once upon a time there was a map. This map belonged to a [pirate/priest/nurse/teacher], who lived in a [swamp/caravan/mansion]. They felt very [sad/angry/fearful] ...'

★ Although this structure is geared towards a murder mystery, it could easily be adjusted to develop a story about an Easter egg hunt or finding buried treasure, for example.

Working with Large Mixed-Ability Groups

The Last Drummer

ORIGINAL SETTING

This project took place in a secondary school working with fifty pupils aged 12 to 17 years who had a variety of needs, from autism spectrum disorders to emotional and behavioural difficulties. In addition to their individual needs, many of the pupils also had English as a second language. The school wanted to encourage cooperation and camaraderie by having pupils from across the school work together for one week, developing a unique theatre piece that would culminate in a performance to family, friends and invited guests.

AIMS

★ To be open to as many pupils as possible (there should be no 'audition' process and pupils should be accepted on their commitment to being involved).

★ To value the pupils' artistic talents and voices in the process and final product (through devising a new play, rather than directing an established script).

★ To raise pupils' expectations of themselves and increase their performance skills (challenges will be created through the introduction of new ways of working and performance skills developed during each workshop, rather than by having specific acting classes).

★ To encourage and promote an ensemble way of working (there should be no lead roles and any that do emerge should be generated organically by the group).

★ To allow the group every chance of succeeding (this does not mean making things easy, but instead, providing a safe working environment for the group to explore, develop and challenge the drama being created).

PREPARATION

In order to achieve these aims and for such a project to succeed, significant time needs to be spent working with both teachers and pupils prior to the workshop week. In addition to confirming the logistics of the project, such as the timetable, support staff and space to be used, such preparation is important for the following reasons:

★ To create enthusiasm in pupils about the project. This can be done through a number of 'taster workshops' that introduce them to drama work.

★ To establish the ground rules for being involved in the project. (Without this, you could end up spending the whole week on nothing but maintaining discipline as the group will need time to develop the necessary skills to succeed at this story-making project.)

★ To discover the topics and themes that are important to the group.

CASE STUDY

Fifty is a very large number to manage for one project. Therefore, three smaller groups were formed to enable the project to run most effectively. The River Tribe was made up of students with moderate learning difficulties, the Desert Tribe was for those with more severe speech and language difficulties, and the Wise Tribe for those pupils needing one-to-one support. As the aim of the project was to bring pupils from across the years together (and keeping those with challenging behaviours engaged and focused throughout the workshops), these groupings worked well for this purpose.

Another important aim of time spent in preparation prior to the workshop week is to get to know the support staff and to set up a code of conduct. This will allow 'play' within the school environment, without staff feeling that existing rules are being challenged, particularly with regard to noise levels.

It is also important that you try to use the support staff's knowledge of the group (such as how individuals may behave in a given situation) when planning your workshops. However, ensuring staff can suspend that knowledge will also give groups the opportunity to work outside of their perceived 'school behaviour' image.

Success of a project such as this can be judged on a number of factors, including the group's commitment to the process (e.g., turning up to rehearsals on time). Feedback from staff not directly involved in the project can also be sought, asking for their comments and observations on how the project has impacted on the wider school environment.

THE STORY STRUCTURE

The story of 'The Last Drummer' created for this project can either be narrated as presented or used as a loose structure for the development of your group's own story.

CASE STUDY

On this project the group were working towards a performance, so the story was originally written as a script. However, the group were not given a written script to work from; instead, one boy took charge of documenting the story through drawings. As he had only been semi-engaged in the early devising process, this task was his idea and became the perfect way of including him fully within the project.

Sample Script – The Last Drummer

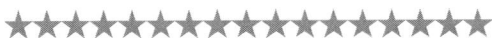

★★★★★★★★★★★★★★★★★

Introduction

The River Tribe must leave their home.

The Desert Tribe need help to survive.

The Wise Tribe send a message into the night trusting the legacy of their ancestors who followed a star.

The River Tribe

Long ago there lived a tribe by the river.

Life was happy.

They would play and eat and whisper secrets to each other.

Smiles abounded as a wedding took place.

People were well.

But one day, things turned bad … Dirty water flowed in the river.

Children would travel great distances to find clean water.

Many would get lost as they tried to find their way home.

Mothers would look for them, holding their young babies close – rocking them.

Fish that once were plentiful were now poison.

People were getting sick … were getting hungry … were getting desperate.

Where there were once smiles there was now anger and concern.

Speculation abounded.

'Someone has poisoned the water.'

'No, it's from everyone using it.'

'All the trees have been cut down and the water is muddy.'

'I'm scared. I'm hungry.'

The leader of the River Tribe stepped forward. He was strong and well respected. Everyone stopped and looked at him as he spoke.

'River people. We have to leave. Our homes. Our friends. Our memories. And find a new home.'

'But were will we go?' asked one member of the Tribe.

The reply came fast. 'We will follow the star.'

The River people began to pack. Began to leave.
They knew their leader was right, but they were still fearful and quietly shared their concerns.
'I don't want to go. I don't.'
'I loved being here.'
'I like eating fish – I might not like other food.'
'It will be a change.'
'We have no choice. We must move.'

And so they did.

The Desert Tribe

The Desert Tribe were happy people. They all laughed and played. And worked to the rhythms of the drums.

Slowly and steadily the drummers would play … beating the rhythm of their tribe.

But one day, things turned bad.
The drums were silent.
No-one had learned the skills of the drum.
They had been too busy with other things … and the knowledge had died.
Soon the work stopped too.

The leader of this tribe was strong. Was respected. He always listened to the concerns of his people.

'Leader we are upset.'

'We are shocked.'

'We don't know what to do.'

During their meeting, a stranger to their land appeared. He brought with him food and water and offered it to the tribal people.

The leader stepped forward to greet him.

'I thank you,' he said 'but it won't help us. Our crops are still dying.'

When in danger, when in darkness, when desperate, there was only one thing this great leader could do.

'I will go and ask the Wise Tribe.'

The Wise Tribe lived in the desert mountains.

The journey was long and the leader had to go alone.

The Wise Tribe

As the leader of the Desert Tribe approached, the oldest of the Wise Tribe spoke.

'We are descendants of the Three Wise Men who followed a star. We have great wisdom. It is wise to help people with things. It is wise to be kind.

Keep your kitchen clean. Don't let the bugs in. And always drink from the toilet.'

Despite being old and wise, they still had a sense of humour!

The Desert Tribe leader stepped forward to ask for advice.

'The drums are silent. My people need help.'

The Wise Tribe whispered to each other.

This was serious. This needed careful thought. This was no time to joke.

After a pause, they had the answer:

'You must send a message into the world. Follow the stars.'

The leader of the Desert people knew that another great journey was ahead of him.

He rested until nightfall and with the blessings of the Wise Tribe set off in search of help.

Following the star.

During the night he walked.

During the day he rested.

He had to succeed. His people needed his help. His people were precious to him.

One night, as the leader was walking, as the leader was doubting, as he was considering turning for home, he saw a shadow ahead.

He stopped. The shadow grew. It took form. It became people.

These people were tired. These people were hungry. These people needed help.

These people were from the River.

Their leader stepped forward and spoke.

'We are travelling to find a new home. We have many skills. We may be of help to you.'

The leader of the Desert people paused before he spoke.

'You are welcome to stay and make this your home, but our tribe also needs help. Do you have a drummer? Someone who could play? Someone who could teach?'

The River people slowly separated as a small figure approached.

He was only a child.

But he could play.

The two tribes were complete.

One had found a new home. The other a drummer. They celebrated together.

Roles & Characters

The following workshop plan was used to develop the storyline for all three tribes, with different choices made by both the River and Desert tribes about life within the village, leadership qualities and how to solve the emerging problems. Although the basic structure was also used for the Wise Tribe, the activities were adapted to suit that group's particular needs.

> ### Adaptations for Groups with Additional Needs
>
> If you have a group with a greater level of needs, instead of looking at pictures for the first activity, you could narrate a story that begins with: 'In the play, you are the Wise Tribe. You are the descendants of three very special wise men who many years ago followed a star…'
>
> The group could then dress in Wise Tribe costumes and have their pictures taken. Now discuss words that describe their characters. Ask the group to practise standing on stage in character, and instead of enacting their roles within the village, the Wise Tribe could demonstrate acts of wisdom and kindness. Each member of the group could decorate a star and each star can be slowly placed on the ground as the group enacts a piece of wise advice or kindness.
>
> A further development could be for you to get into role as someone asking them for advice, so their story drama of acting wisely, performing their ritual and giving advice all come together.

Props & Materials

★ A selection of evocative pictures of rivers/deserts

★ Blank paper (A3 size preferable)

★ Water-based marker pens

★ Craft materials such as scissors, glitter, string

★ A selection of music and/or musical instruments (to reflect the chosen picture environments)

★ Sticky notes

★ Props or costume to denote each tribe

Story-Building Activities

Activity: Looking At Pictures

★ Give out paper, pens and copies of either the desert or river pictures.

For any pupils with visual impairment, pictures could be replaced by sensory representations of the various locations. For example, sandpaper, an oil burner or incense sticks, dried leaves or other foliage, furry material or evocative music could all help to stimulate the senses for a desert environment.

★ Either as a whole group or in supported smaller groups, ask everyone to brainstorm and record words and/or phrases that describe what they see and imagine from these images. Questions to help stimulate the group's imagination could include:

– What colours do you see?

– What is in the photo (trees, sand, camels, etc.). What is not in the photo (just outside the image or possibly hiding somewhere in it)?

– How do you feel when looking at this image?

– How would you feel if you were in this picture?

– What do you think you could smell?

– What type of animals would live here?

Note: Ensure you tell the group that there are no right or wrong answers and that it is fine if the different groups come up with the same words, as it shows how important these words are. The aim is to create a visual collage reflecting their thoughts and ideas on the images presented, helping to build belief in an imagined world.

Groups might then wish to create a tactile display inspired by their newly discovered environment.

Activity: Movement & Ritual

★ Ask the group to choose a word or phrase from their created list.

★ Individually or in pairs, ask everyone to develop a *repeatable* movement (and possibly sound) to represent it.

Note: This abstract concept could be quite foreign to some groups. Again reiterate that there is no 'right' way of doing this and the movements can be as literal or poetic as they like.

Demonstrate and support this activity as much as possible. For example, to represent the word 'water' pupils might come up with the action of swimming, bathing, drinking, or just moving about the space with a fluid motion.

★ Now show the movements to the rest of the group and encourage demonstrators to be as slow as possible with their movements. This will not only encourage physical discipline and awareness but will enhance the theatrical ritual being created.

★ Ask the groups to simultaneously perform their own movements to music to create a large tribal ritual.

For groups who need less support, link up two individuals (or pairs) and ask them to combine their movements. If possible, add the following staging progression:

– Simultaneously perform their original movements to music.

– At a chosen signal slowly find their link-up partners and then start performing (together) their second combined movement.

– At next signal, go back to their original individual movements.

★ When finished, ask the group to sit down as you read out their chosen keywords or phrases, (topping and tailing with a sentence such as, 'We are the *River/Desert* tribe') to create the first part of their story. For example:

"We are the River Tribe. Water flows. People drink. Villagers swim. They look out for danger. They fish. Swimming. Blue. Cold. Deep. We are the River People."

Activity: Discovering the Inhabitants

★ Once the environment has been explored, discuss with the group about the type of people who might live there and record these answers on paper too. Questions to prompt the discussion (and their subsequent actions) could include:

- What type of people might live here?

- What would they wear?

- What would they eat?

- Where would they sleep?

- How would they get around?

- What do they do for fun?

- Do they have a particular job in the village?

★ Tell the group that you will now be asking them to take on the role of an inhabitant of the tribe. Ask them to think about their role/job/task in this *happy* village.

Note: It is important that they start from a happy place, otherwise the drama will have nowhere to go. If the tribes are unhappy to begin with, what weight will the introduced problem hold?

★ With a partner, get them to practise their role/job/task with each other before sharing with the group. Ask them to precede these demonstrations with the sentence, 'In the Desert Tribe I...'

CASE STUDY

It is important to accept any answer and work it in to the developing story if you possibly can. In one group a pupil was obsessed with James Bond. We therefore had a tribal spy who had an extremely important job of protecting the village. Another boy was intent on being an American soldier, whose character became vital to the story through visiting the dying tribe and offering short-term help. It was during this activity that the tribal leader also emerged.

★ As with the words and movements generated by the pictures, ask the group to repeat their actions simultaneously around the room, accompanied by music appropriate to the chosen environment. These movements should be at a *regular* speed to demonstrate a happy village life.

★ Stop the action and ask the group 'How do you greet each other?' Get them to develop greetings within the tribe. Possibly extend by asking, 'How do you greet other tribes/villages?'

CASE STUDY

An amazing greeting developed when one tribe, upon meeting another, was initially wary and gave out subtle movements of friendship, while displaying acts of strength. The whole ritual was quite complex, very primitive and took us completely by surprise!

★ To further encourage village life, ask the group what sort of things the tribe might celebrate. These could include weddings, a harvest or the waking of the sun. As a whole group, develop this celebratory ritual. You might want to dress up in a special costume, paint faces or hands and actually cook some food as part of this celebration.

CASE STUDY

We had a wedding ceremony and as well as enacting the ceremony (incorporating variations from different multi-cultural traditions), we played the game 'Present Giving' in which imaginary gifts are given. It is up to the person receiving the gift to name what it is, although the 'gift giver' can help to prompt by pretending to carry a gift that is large and heavy, or small and delicate.

★ To finish this activity the group could draw around their hands and, in the outline of each finger, record an aspect of village life. For example, their role within the village, their celebration, a symbol to represent their name and so forth. These 'Hand Print Images' could then form part of their tactile collage.

Activity: The Leader

★ Narrate the following to the group, 'Our tribe has a leader. His/her role is very special…'

★ Ask the tribal leader to stand in front of the group.

Note: If no leader has emerged by this time (or if he/she is unwilling to stand in front of the group) you could use an adaptation of the 'Role on the Wall' technique by drawing the outline of a person on a large piece of paper. Alternatively you might like to ask for a volunteer to act as the leader, or take on the role yourself.

> **ROLE ON THE WALL**
>
> The outline of a person is drawn on a large piece of paper. The group then brainstorm words to describe the character and these are written inside the image. Extensions to this basic strategy can include:
>
> ★ Recording the character's thoughts about themselves within the outline.
>
> ★ Recording what other characters think or say about the character on the outside of the image.
>
> ★ Using different colours or pictures to represent different emotions.

Discuss the following with the group:

★ What do we want the leader of our tribe to be like? For example, strong, tall, brave, clever.

★ What is important for a leader to be able to do? For example, hunt, fight, be calm, be able to stop arguments.

★ Write the answers to each question on sticky notes and attach them to the leader.

CASE STUDY

It turned out that the boy who emerged as the natural leader of the Desert Tribe was actually quite withdrawn and often disruptive within the school environment. School staff were initially wary about allowing him to have the responsibility of being the group's leader, yet throughout the workshops he was a natural and the rest of the tribe treated him with the greatest respect. This proved to be a good example of the differences between perceived behaviour within the school environment and behaviour within a safe dramatic play environment.

★ Review these words with the group, and discuss with the chosen leader their thoughts on what is important for a tribe leader. Ask the leader to choose the three words from each list that they believe to be the most important.

Note: Allowing the leaders to choose for themselves the most important qualities, rather than have the group as a whole do so, can be a useful activity to refer back to should the leader's attitude change. This can be especially important if you are working with a group who have behavioural difficulties.

★ Re-introduce this leader to the group using narration and 'Teacher-In-Role' (TIR). For example, 'Desert Tribe, I welcome this leader. She is wise. She is strong. She is patient. She can cook. She can protect us. She can find water. She is our leader. The leader of the Desert Tribe.'

★ The group could develop a greeting or small ritual for their leader, such as a bow, or a salute and a cheer.

Note: 'Teacher-In-Role' (TIR) is not about displaying exceptional acting talent; instead it is about demonstrating commitment to the drama or story being created. When done well it is completely selfless, honouring the work being created and encouraging excellence in the participants.

Activity: What Went Wrong?

★ Ask the group to repeat their happy village life actions. Once finished, introduce a dilemma facing the village through either narration or TIR.

Note: You might need to forewarn the group that you are going to go into role, pretending to be a character from their village. Tell them that they will need to listen carefully to see what information they can pick up and that you will be expecting them to answer or join in the drama 'in-role' themselves.

> The dilemma facing the village could be anything. However, from the work developed by the group so far, you may find that a problem has already presented itself. If not, you could start the introduction and then ask the group, 'What is the problem facing our village/tribe?'

> If working in-role, encourage the group to respond in-role. For example, refer to certain people and say, 'I know you've been personally affected by this problem, would you like to tell us about it?' (If they do not, acknowledge this by saying something like: 'I know it's been a difficult experience, so don't worry if you're not able to tell us.' Often this will encourage another pupil to share an experience.)

> If you are not confident working 'in-role' then you may wish to prompt a discussion by asking the group how they think this dilemma might personally affect the people of the village.

★ Once the problem has been explored, drop role and ask the group to work in pairs or small groups to show an image of how this dilemma has affected their village character personally.

★ Start with a still image which could 'come to life' for 30 seconds before freezing again.

★ As an extension you might like to create a 'dream-like' state with these images by asking the group to explore the following dramatic conventions within their 30 second scenes:

  – Repetition (with both movement and sound/words/phrases)

  – Freeze-frame and rewind

- Slow-motion

- Sounds (both inner thoughts and words or sounds to create mood and atmosphere)

- Mirroring actions

★ As the group perform their still images or 'dream-like' actions simultaneously around the room, add appropriate music to provide a wonderful contrast to their original *happy* tribal state.

CASE STUDY

The following examples were created by the Desert and River Tribes. The Desert Tribe's problem was introduced via narration from their collected words and drama work, while for the River Tribe it was through the role of a 'concerned villager'.

'Desert Tribe, our desert was an Oasis. Minerals could be extracted from the flowers that grew here and we never had to travel far for water. We built sandcastles and lived in caves.

Now we are lonely, bored, isolated and lost.

Quicksand steals the flowers and we feel stranded. Someone must tell the leader.

He is wise, strong and patient. The tribe looks to him for guidance but they are still fearful. They are scared, thirsty and sad.

The drums don't sound. There is no-one to play them. They stand unused.'

'River people, I am worried. For many years now the river has supported our tribe. We have drunk the water, bathed and played along the banks. But things have changed. The river is dirty and we suffer.

What was once a happy, relaxed and proud land is now angry, destructive and lonely.

We have sacrificed.

Children drown in the water.

Our sacred shelters of gold are now muddy ruins.

We have nothing to eat.

Food that was once in abundance is now gone in our lifeless river.

We were hunters. We were proud. We lived by the rhythms of the river.

Our traditions are dying.'

Activity: Rumour & Gossip

★ After each group has chosen the problem facing their tribe and examined how it affects them personally, ask each person to choose either a word, short phrase or sound that represents how they feel about living in this tribe now.

★ Introduce groups to the activity through narration. For example, 'Nobody knew quite what to do. They talked and whispered to each other. Rumour and gossip was everywhere. No-one knew what to believe. As the leader walked about the tribe he/she heard what was being said.'

★ Ask the group to form a line and to whisper their chosen word or phrase over and over as the leader of the tribe walks along the line. Guide the tribe by asking them to repeat their word/phrase (the gossip) using different emotions e.g., sad, angry, excited, concerned.

If members of the group have speech and language difficulties, photographs could be taken of them acting out the 'What Went Wrong' activity which could then be presented to the leader. Alternatively words, phrases or sounds could be recorded on personal communication devices which could then build into a wonderful cacophony of sounds.

★ Once the leader has completed the walk, ask him/her about what they heard and to repeat some of the words or phrases coming from the tribe. (You might also like to repeat this activity with other members of the group taking on the role of the leader.) Ask how they felt when hearing these comments. You may need to demonstrate this first and assist the leader as they walk down the line.

The Decision

Now that the problem has been decided, a solution needs to be found. Again, depending on the problem, a solution might have already presented itself. There are numerous strategies to help move the story/drama forward. See 'The Sleeping Boy' for further development ideas that can lead on from this workshop plan including:

★ Creating tribal artwork such as cave paintings or pottery with images of the outcome.

★ Developing a musical ritual with movement, sound, materials, speeches, prayers.

★ Going on a shared journey.

CASE STUDY

The River Tribe decided to leave their home so they each packed a bag, deciding what they would be able to take on the journey ahead, and sharing their thoughts on leaving.

The Desert Tribe decided to send their leader off to visit the Wise Tribe for advice and, to help describe his journey, the group used a large piece of brown material. They created mountains (by standing underneath it and stretching up) and wind storms (shaking the material violently) while I narrated the leader's journey. The group also stamped a rhythm that increased in tempo and volume before coming to a 'stop' to signal the end of the journey.

FURTHER DEVELOPMENT

Instead of writing the story down, the group might like to storyboard their developing drama, either documenting each stage of the story on a separate piece of paper or creating the completed story on one large sheet.

Working with Young Children & Families or Carers

The Sleeping Boy

ORIGINAL SETTING

This workshop plan was part of a ten-week project that aimed to develop original stories through drama with 5 to 11 year olds with learning difficulties and their families or carers. Each workshop lasted for two hours, with a 15 minute break, and took place in the basement of a local museum. The room was well equipped with coloured mats, beanbags and musical instruments. The space could also be split into two distinct sections (which became invaluable as the project developed).

Participants were recruited from the local community and nearby SEN schools. Many of the families had refugee status and English as an additional language. To aid with recruitment, a taster workshop was held three weeks prior to the start of the project. This was designed to give staff the chance to meet those already signed up and to give other potential participants the chance to find out what the project was all about.

The taster workshop was invaluable as it revealed the vast range of ages and needs amongst the potential participants. Ages ranged from 2 to 14 years, with siblings as young as four months old. The needs ranged from mild autistim to more profound physical and learning difficulties. There were also a number of young people who were extremely 'space sensitive' and needed ongoing support simply to stay in the room.

Support

As well as the dramatherapist and story-maker, there were five volunteer assistants, some of whom were trainee teachers. Parents were strongly encouraged to stay during the sessions, not only to provide additional support but also to explore new and creative ways to engage with their child. The project was intended to be family-orientated (hence the invitation for siblings to participate) and so it was hoped that the majority of parents would stay throughout.

Despite efforts to encourage family inclusion some parents chose not to participate at all during the taster workshop. Their absence had a big impact as providing one-to-one care for the unaccompanied children was extremely demanding and slowed down the story-making process. Some children also found being left alone quite difficult. To cope with this parents were encouraged to remain with their child for a set time during the early stages of the project. Then, over the period the project, they left their child alone for a little longer each week until the child was happy to be left for the whole session.

Group Size & Inclusion Policy

Originally, the project involved fifteen children but as the weeks passed the group settled down to a core of approximately twelve. This meant that space became available for those on a waiting list. It is always a challenge to introduce new people part-way through a project and so new participants were only accepted for the first three weeks. Had the project been longer than ten weeks, it may have been possible to extend this period. However, it is important to realise the impact that newcomers will have on the rest of the group, especially those sensitive to change. It is useful to put an inclusion policy in place from the outset which states clearly the point at which new members will no longer be accepted.

Attendance & The Space

Attendance and punctuality can often be a problem, especially when a project is free of charge. Many of the children arrived late for this project and this had a big impact on the group as a whole. As well as missing out on the story work being developed, the latecomers often found it difficult to settle as they had missed the welcome rituals.

To overcome this problem it was decided that the first half-hour of the workshop would occur in one part of the space, with any latecomers being asked to remain in a separate area where various multi-sensory items were provided to keep them engaged until they could be welcomed in.

CASE STUDY

The area outside the main workshop room was turned into multi-sensory space with materials, beanbags, instruments, puppets and other toys, supported by the dramatherapist. This was beneficial for two reasons. First, it provided a creative time-out space for children who found it difficult to remain in the main room. It also allowed latecomers to feel immediately engaged and welcome before being introduced into the story-making space at an appropriate point. This second space became a crucial element in the project as it allowed the story-making to continue without major disruption. There were also times when the story-making migrated out of the main room and into the multi-sensory space so that those in the outside room felt more included.

It became clear through ongoing re-evaluation of the project's structure that the process of finding and developing each participant's 'voice' would take time and patience. Creating an environment that would encourage and develop each person's skills and imagination, as well as take on board their communication and learning needs was very challenging. However, with increasing knowledge and understanding of each individual, a positive and safe space was eventually created, where the group felt able to take risks and share their ideas. This, as well as ongoing communication between all staff involved, resulted in a successful project where a truly meaningful story was created with the group.

THE STORY STRUCTURE

The story of 'The Sleeping Boy' is one of a group of stories built around an imaginary village, inhabited by the 'Drawn People'. The concept of the Drawn People came about during the initial taster session when the group were exploring the idea of clay, gardens, rocks and the earth through images, sounds and colour. One young boy, after looking at some photographs of rocks, made a link with cave drawings and the people who drew them, hence the Drawn People were born. The following workshop was explored over several sessions and developed into a grand adventure, however, it all began when one of the participants was tired and wanted to go to sleep… he became the 'Sleeping Boy'.

Props & Materials

★ Gym mats or squares of carpet

★ Selection of music and/or musical instruments

★ Large piece of brown fabric

★ Tables and fabric with which to create a 'tunnel'

★ Collection of 'bouncing' spiders (can be made from cardboard and elastic)

★ Vampire bat (or alternative) toy or costume

★ A star

★ Crocodile soft toy, puppet or costume (optional)

★ Blank paper (A3 size preferable)

★ Water-based marker pens

★ Bird (or other creature) puppet

★ Large paper 'eye' (can be created by the group)

★ Torch

★ Different coloured objects/scarves (optional)

★ Length of rope

★ Shawl or other prop for the Enchantress character

★ Large carpet or piece of material

PREPARATION

You will need to develop the group's belief in an imagined world (of their choice) prior to starting the workshop. This can be done in a number of ways:

★ Look at pictures related to the world. For example, a city, a wood or a room.

★ Develop a movement activity in which the group walk through the imagined environment as you narrate the world around them.

★ Ask group members to draw an object that might be found in that world.

★ Create still images of life within that world.

★ Discuss with the group how the imagined world is different from their own.

Note: See the activities in 'The Last Drummer' for a detailed breakdown of creating an imagined world, as the same activities were used in the preliminary stages to create the village of the Drawn People. See also Handout 16.

Sample Script –
Extract from The Story of the Sleeping Boy

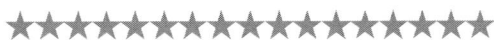

★★★★★★★★★★★★★★★★★★★★★★★

Everyone in the village had a job, had a role, had a task to perform.

And every job and every role and every task was completed with the greatest care.

It was somebody's job to wash the clothes. The smelly, ripped and ragged clothes – from swimming and riding and hunting – needed to be cleaned.

It was somebody's job to manage the camels. To brush them, and feed them – with dried grasses and left-over vegetables – and saddle them ready for an immediate journey that might need to be taken.

The village even had a chocolate maker. He made the creamiest, tastiest, darkest chocolate – as dark as the clay the Drawn People saw around them in the caves and the mountains – which was wrapped in delicate paper and put in the shade to cool.

But there was one task in the village that was never quite understood. It was always somebody's job to sleep.

For as long as the Drawn People could remember, there was always a sleeping boy in the village. He would sleep for a whole year and the moment he awoke, someone else would suddenly sleep.

Many had tried to wake him.

They tried yelling.
They tried singing.
They even tried tickling him.

But until that year was up, the sleeping boy would sleep.

There had been a rumour of a spell. Perhaps from a Witch. Or an Enchantress. Or a Queen.

But no-one had ever seen. No-one had ever heard. Until one day …

… they decided to go and find out …

The Drawn People did not want to go on this quest without the necessary skills, so they chose three of the bravest villagers to plan the training.

For those that wished to enter the training, there were three tasks that needed to be learned, that needed to be practised, that needed to be perfected.

The first skill needed was using a sword.

A diagonal slash down.

    A vertical slash forward.

        A strong throw through the air.

The second skill needed was in making a potion.

Collecting the venom of a snake.

    Stirring it in the mud until it bubbled.

        Keeping it safe in a stopped-up bottle.

The third skill needed was magic.

When fighting a Witch, an Enchantress, a Queen – magic is needed.

The Drawn People used the magic of the Mountains. Pulling on the electric shocks of the rocks the Drawn People would collect it in their hands.

    Building up the power.

        Holding it in until the electricity built to its maximum level.

           Releasing it towards the target – SPELL SHOCK!

The greatest care was needed when using SPELL SHOCK!

Held too long in the hands and it would affect the caster.

Released too early and it would not hit the target.

This skill took the longest to master.

Those of the Drawn People going on the quest trained for days.

Day and night. Over and over.

Until all the skills were learned.

When the training was complete, the village gathered round.

It was a day of rejoicing.

      It was a day of celebration.

            It was also a day of sadness. A quest can be dangerous.

The Drawn People who were not going performed a ritual. For protection. For the group.

Each person brought something new, something special, something secret to the sacred circle.

A star was given.

A star that had been caught by climbing to the highest peak of the highest mountain.

It was given for light. To help the group when in darkness – when in danger.

As the star was given, the Drawn People of the village began to chant:

Drawn People, Drawn People we will cast a spell.

Drawn People, Drawn People we will cast it well.

Drawn People, Drawn People we will have no rest.

Drawn People, Drawn People protection for your quest.

Sitting on her throne in her cave – a cave with eyes that were open –
the Witch, the Enchantress, the Queen, called her spiders to her.

'The Drawn People are coming' she said.

'Don't let them through. Alert me when you're done.'

STORY-BUILDING ACTIVITIES

The Problem

Once the group have established their imagined world (and explored their roles within the village/community) introduce the following problem through narration and discussion. For example:

"For as long as the village could remember, there had been a sleeping boy. Nothing could wake him. Over the years, many of the villagers had tried to wake him up, but he continued to sleep..."

Activity: Wake Up

In this 'wake-up' game individuals can take on either the role of the sleeping boy (or girl), or a villager trying to wake him up. The only rule of the game is that the 'wakers' are not allowed to touch the sleeping boy.

Strategies to wake the boy can include sound orchestras, imaginary buckets of water, large feathers or wafted material. The person pretending to be the sleeping boy must try to ignore all efforts, as they try to continue sleeping. If they move or are 'awakened' swap over.

To aid in the swap-over of sleeping boys, and avoid potential difficulties, narrate the following:

"After one year of sleeping, the boy would automatically wake up. However, just as he awoke, another would suddenly ... fall asleep!"

> ### CASE STUDY
>
> This game helped to engage the boy who initially created the role. He was so proud that his actions had been developed, incorporated and accepted by the group that he started to oversee others who took on the part of the sleeping boy, waiting with glee until it was his turn to once again go back to sleep.

Questions to help prompt exploration of the problem of the sleeping boy could include:

★ Why do you think this boy is sleeping?

★ Do you think it was an Enchantress who cast a spell or gave him poison?

★ If it was an Enchantress, why do you think she cast this spell?

Note: This can lead into an interesting exploration of what motivates people to do 'bad' things. Try introducing a 'hot-seat' activity with someone in-role as the Enchantress (or alternative), being questioned by the group as to her motives. This could be a member of staff or one of the group. This activity could develop into a valuable discussion on bullying, friendship and behaviour.

For pupils with more complex learning needs, it could be that the drama revolves around bringing in a new character to create a magic spell that will wake up the sleeping boy. The quest could involve having each 'brave' participant enter her cave to ask for help.

The Quest

To introduce the idea of going on a quest, narrate the following:

> *"Before embarking on their quest to find the Enchantress responsible for the curse of the sleeping boy, those chosen needed to prepare for their journey."*

Activity: Preparing for the Quest

Discuss with the group how they might prepare for their journey, for example:

★ What to take?

Develop a mime activity in which everyone packs their own belongings for the journey. Alternatively you could use an actual backpack or suitcase and ask the group to draw pictures of what they might need for the trip, and put these in the bag.

★ What skills are needed?

Ask the group to think about special skills that might be needed when going on a quest. Working as individuals, pairs or small groups (with guided support) develop these special skills to teach to the rest of the group. Each skill should have a movement and/or sound that the rest of the group can copy.

CASE STUDY

Our group came up with sword skills, potion-making and a magic spell called 'Spell Shock'. As a final test to assess whether the group were ready for the quest, we adapted the 'Compass Game' (in which people have to run to parts of the room labelled North, South, East or West at different commands). In this version, points of the room were labelled with the different skills, so when 'Spell Shock' was called the group had to go to the red mats and perform the movement and sound for that particular skill.

One pupil was not interested in going on the quest or developing a skill and so he became the official 'judge', and relished his role when it came to assessing the rest of the group's competence in the 'skills test'.

Activity: The Leaving Ritual

★ To add weight and importance to the drama/story, you might like to develop a leaving ritual organised by the village. Collect the group into a circle and narrate the following:

"Before embarking on their quest, the villagers gathered together to perform their ancient ritual; a ritual of protection that would guard over those going on this very important quest..."

★ Discuss with the group what this ritual might be (again, individuals, pairs or small groups could develop their own part of the ritual). Whatever is developed, encourage the group to present their part of the ritual in slow motion and repeat it at least twice (you may even want to dim the lights or spend time decorating the room).

Ideas for the ritual could involve one or more of the following:

– A song (an original composition or one that the group knows well, but not one that has previously been used in the sessions)

– A dance or movement piece (this could be accompanied by another group playing musical instruments or an appropriate piece of music)

– The telling of a story

– The passing around of a sacred object from the village (with a narration or discussion as to why it is sacred and special)

– The giving of goodbye or protection gifts to those going on the quest

---

CASE STUDY

On this project, the Leaving Ritual was developed with those in the group who needed more one-to-one support and was performed to the rest of the group. It provided a wonderful way of incorporating this group into the story and allowed them to be leaders for part of the session.

★ End the ritual with the group lying down and pretending to go to sleep.

Note: For more able groups you could 'thought-track' their dreams by asking them to reflect on the events to come. Walk among the group and when you tap a person on the shoulder, they could whisper either a word or sentence which expresses how they are feeling about the journey ahead.

CREATING ENVIRONMENTS & JOURNEYS

There are various strategies you could use for creating an imagined journey or environment. You might like to prepare one or two ideas or environments to help kick-start the group, or have a number of sensory props standing by for whatever the group decides to create.

Strategies for Creating an Environment

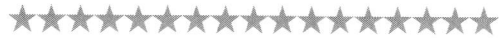

★★★★★★★★★★★★★★★★★★★★

★ *Narration* – usually done by the drama/story leader with the group listening as you describe the details of an imaginary environment.

★ *Teacher In Role* (TIR) – an extension of Narration and extremely effective for introducing new or established characters into an environment and helping to guide the group's ideas (See the chapter 'Staying in Control' for more on this strategy).

★ *Mimed Movement* – often done in association with narration or music. For example: 'The group came to a land with rocks and cactus scattered everywhere. It was very dangerous and they had to move in single file, making sure they held on to each other as they walked slowly through...'

★ *Soundscape* – ask the group to create the sounds for the environment with their voices (including electronic communication devices), bodies and/or musical instruments. You can then physically guide the volume and speed of this soundscape. For example, slowly raising and lowering your arms to increase or decrease the volume, pointing to individuals to either silence them or have them stand out, or spinning your arms in a circle to have the group speed up. Some group members might also like to have a go at being the 'conductor'. This soundscape could be recorded and played back to the group.

★ *Obstacle Courses* – wonderfully effective in the right space and can be incorporated into a physical education class. Ask the group to help you design the obstacle course (and even demonstrate how to manoeuvre through it). Benches, mats, hoops, rope, tunnels, long pieces of material, lycra or elastic can all be used, with the group encouraging each other make it through.

★ *Creating a Den* – a decorated space, such as an ultra-violet room, classroom or even just a series of tables covered with sheets. This could also involve the exploration of sensory elements such as smells (incense sticks, scented oils on tissue, or jars containing different scented objects), touch (discovering objects in sand) or taste (exploring different fruits perhaps). Entering into the den can be narrated, for example:

> *"The group decided to camp for the night. As they made their way into the tents each made their own special discovery ..."*

When they emerge they could show the rest of the group what they have found.

★ *Playing/Adapting Games* (see the chapter 'Breaking Down the Drama Game' for a description of these and other games).

A game such as 'Camera Blink' (Handout 8) could be used to discover a new location. 'Count 21' (Handout 9) might be adapted as a test, with the group not able to continue on their journey until they are successful, while a version of 'Go If' (Handout 11) could be used to set up camp for the night, ensuring the group has all the necessary equipment.

DEVELOPING A QUEST

The following quest from 'The Sleeping Boy' story uses a number of the different strategies mentioned.

Activity: The Tunnel

★ Introduce a tunnel via narration. This not only establishes a location, but gives instructions on how to move through it.

> "The group came to a tunnel. It was dark and spooky and was only wide enough for one person to go through at a time."

★ Allow the group to spend some time creating an obstacle course, and introduce the concept of the tunnel being full of spiders. This can lead to a discussion about what people should do if they encounter the spiders.

★ Now develop a game. One by one the group must make their way through the tunnel as the toy or cardboard spiders are 'bounced' above them, covering the exit. The rule of the game is that the person in the tunnel must stay motionless while the spiders are bouncing. To safely escape from the tunnel, develop a count in which the spiders bounce for a count of five and then rest for a count of five, allowing enough time for people to get through without the spiders seeing them.

★ Once through, allow the group to rest. Give someone in the group a set of imaginary binoculars and ask them to see what is up ahead.

Activity: A Swamp

★ While sitting down, ask the group to create a soundscape to help establish the swamp. From the sounds created, think about how it might feel to be in the swamp, e.g., quite spooky and dangerous or friendly and light.

★ Create another obstacle course using mats to jump on (acting as rocks jutting out of the murky water). A large piece of brown material can be used as 'mud' for people to move beneath or sit on as support workers drag the material across the floor.

★ Before the group set off, use narration to establish the character of a watchful Vampire Bat. Then as the first brave volunteer starts to make their way across the swamp, the Vampire Bat (TIR) can swoop down and confront them! This bat (or alternative) could also be in the form of a soft toy that swoops down over the group.

★ Discuss in the group how to combat the attacking Vampire Bat, before the group set out across the swamp again.

CASE STUDY

During the discussion on how to combat the Vampire Bat, the group remembered a 'Star of Protection' that had been given to them during the Leaving Ritual. They decided that this star would be held aloft as the Vampire Bat swooped, effectively using the light to scare him away. This was a clever connection that the group made entirely for themselves, and we then practised using the star to frighten the bat away. Once we were ready, another child decided that he would play the Vampire Bat and consequently had great fun screeching away from the light of the star.

CASE STUDY

During our journey across the swamp, the character of a crocodile appeared from under the water. As the group were escaping to the opposite bank, one child suddenly mimed falling into the water and being swallowed up.

Rather than dismiss this development, it was incorporated into the drama. The group had to decide whether to risk the dangers of the swamp to rescue him, or to continue on their quest. The discussion included a debate on whether the boy would still be alive or not and whether or not it was worth risking the lives of others to save him. A secret vote was taken to decide on what to do.

Ultimately the decision was left to the leader and they decided to move forward on their quest, but spent one minute in silence for their fallen comrade.

As for the boy who instigated all this by being swallowed, he sat watching the entire process from the other side of the room and once they had finished their silent memorial, he was 'de-roled' and brought back into the group to help create the next part of the quest.

Activity: Enchanted Wood

★ Narration was used establish the wood and its possible dangers, with guidance on how to move through it.

"The group found themselves on the edge of a dark wood. Tall trees were everywhere. As they moved slowly through the wood they were certain the trees were moving too..."

★ Play an adaptation of the game 'Grandmother's Footsteps' with half of the group being cast as trees. The rest must try and move from one side of the room to the other without being caught or surrounded by the 'trees'. If the trees are looked at directly they have to freeze. You may need to take a little time to demonstrate this and perhaps hold some practise runs.

★ As more and more of the group become entangled in the trees, a bird puppet (TIR with puppet) can be introduced to scare the trees away. This puppet can be used to not only rescue the group but to provide information on how to find the Enchantress. It can also give the group a useful opportunity to recap on their adventure so far.

Activity: A Cave

Thanks to the information provided by the bird puppet and suggestions from the group, it can be discovered that the Enchantress lives in a cave. This cave is guarded by a magical eye and it is only possible to enter the cave when the eye closes on the night of the full moon.

★ Get the group to help you create a cave and a large paper eye that can close (or it could be made using a body sculpture by the group). The cave entrance can also have music or sound playing in the background to help set the mood.

★ Stick the large eye above or beside the doorway to the cave and have the group gather outside to watch as the eye slowly closes. Use music to accompany the dimming of the lights and the light of a torch to sweep over the group. When the eye is closed, everyone can sneak through the doorway.

★ Once inside, the group must answer a question in order to proceed, such as naming their favourite colour. This can be staged by having the group 'penned in' by a circle of chairs. They are not allowed out of the circle until they have answered their question.

★ Once the questions have been answered, move everyone onto mats to hear the narration of the next part of the cave. For example:

"The group found themselves on the edge of a steep cliff.
There was only enough room to move in single file and they had to
move slowly to avoid slipping ..."

★ Set up a rope balance by placing a length of rope along the floor. The group must walk along the rope, balancing one foot in front of the other until they reach the other side, and find themselves trapped back in a circle of chairs or wrapped in a piece of material, just as the Enchantress appears!

Note: This exercise can be adapted for those with limited mobility by passing a rope through the group, entangling everyone. For extra drama, narrate the danger of a passing light (possibly the watchful eye of the Enchantress). Therefore, whenever the torchlight shines on someone they must freeze!

MANAGING AN ENCOUNTER

As the quest is leading towards meeting the Enchantress (who is responsible for making the boy sleep in the village) develop the following progression to help anyone who might be uncertain about meeting this potentially frightening character.

First, ask everyone to help you create the look of the character by choosing which items of clothing she might wear and deciding how she might move and speak. As each decision is made, model it for the group before adopting the role fully as part of the drama (using TIR). Introducing the character slowly and empowering the group with its creation, can help to minimise any potential distress.

Activity: Meeting the Enchantress

As the group are sitting 'trapped', the Enchantress appears and dances around the group reciting:

> "Drawn People, Drawn People I will cast a spell.
> Drawn People, Drawn People, and my spell will smell!
> Drawn People, Drawn People so that you can't tell...
> Drawn People, Drawn People you will sleep quite well."

Drop the role and ask the group the following questions:

★ Why do you think the Enchantress made the spell?

★ How do you think the villagers could break the spell?

★ Would this help them to escape?

Note: Try out any suggestions as many times as necessary. Ultimately the group should be successful in their escape, but the number of ideas that are tried before they succeed is at your discretion.

CASE STUDY

A wonderful combination of ideas emerged during our discussion. It had been established early on that there was an ice-cream maker in the village. It was decided to offer ice-cream to the Enchantress. However, it would be laced with poison... A volunteer was then chosen to approach the Enchantress and it was their job to convince her to eat the ice-cream. The group took great glee in watching the Enchantress slowly eat the ice-cream and the poison having its effect on her. There were cheers as she slowly sank to the floor.

RECAPPING & HONOURING THE ADVENTURE

Activity: The Magic Carpet

Place a large carpet (or piece of material) on the floor and narrate the following:

"The Enchantress was defeated. Suddenly the cave magically disappeared and the group found themselves floating high above the woods …"

Assemble the group on the Magic Carpet, play some music and ask them to point out moments and landmarks from their adventure as they fly home.

Activity: Arriving Home

On arrival get the group into a circle for a welcome-home celebration. This could involve a party (complete with food), a celebration dance or the playing of a game.

CASE STUDY

We decided to play the game 'Copy Me' in which everyone stands in a circle while some music is played. In slow motion, a chosen individual starts a movement for the rest of the group to copy. Ensure you go around the circle so that everyone has the chance to lead the group if they wish.

At the end of the celebration, place 'The Sleeping Boy' in the centre of the room, guiding him with the following narration:

"At the end of the celebration, the village gathered around the sleeping boy and slowly watched as he yawned, stretched his arms, blinked his eyes and stood up. The village cheered as the spell was finally broken."

This 'waking up' activity can also be done with the whole group taking on the role of the Sleeping Boy, rather than just one individual.

Ask the group to retell the story of their adventure. This can be done verbally or through drawings.

FURTHER DEVELOPMENT

To help reinforce the adventure, the group could create artwork or a visual timeline of their adventure. You could interview individuals as they recall moments from their quest and record a sound collage of their responses for people to listen to.

Taking photographs of the group throughout their story-making process can also be used to help reinforce the work created. (NB Ensure that you obtain any necessary permission to do so.)

Working with an Unplanned Change of Venue

The Disappearing Monkeys

ORIGINAL SETTING

From time to time the routine or plans for your group can change unexpectedly and with little notice. The following story was developed due to the regular workshop space for 'The Sleeping Boy' being unavailable one day.

If you do encounter such a disruption to the routine of a regular group, be aware that your participants will have become familiar and comfortable in their regular space and with their regular timetable and that this could prove distressing and distracting to some members of the group. You may well find that you have to spend time adjusting to the new surroundings and as a consequence have a much reduced period of time in which to work.

However, even with reduced time you will find that you can still build on your story from previous sessions and work on activities which can be developed further once your normal routine is re-established.

Try to minimise any confusion and distress by:

★ Continuing to use your regular 'meet and greet' activities.

★ Including as many familiar elements in the new room as possible, such as recognised cushions, instruments and props.

★ Providing extra support staff where possible for those individuals who might have an adverse reaction to the change.

★ Allowing extra time for settling and recapping, and don't worry should there only be a short amount of focused work within the session.

★ Turning the 'journey to a new room' into part of the story adventure, such as 'travelling to a different part of the jungle'.

Props & Materials

You will need:

★ Bubbles

★ Balloons

★ Some long blue material, parachute or large piece of lycra (optional)

★ Three 'monkeys' (such as soft toys or picture representations)

★ Gym mats or squares of carpet

★ Water mist spray

★ Some curtain netting

★ A collection of sea creatures and/or objects such as shells.

★ A selection of instruments related to water e.g., ocean drums, shakers, rain sticks

★ Recorded sea music/sounds of waves and waterfalls (or music suggestive of this)

★ Water creatures and forest/jungle puppets (optional)

★ Shells, stones and other sea/water-related objects

★ A willing teaching assistant!

Sample Script – The Disappearing Monkeys

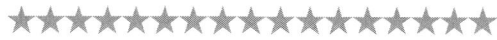

★★★★★★★★★★★★★★★★★★

We are the Drawn People and we live among the rocks in the Mountains.

Water sprays out of the rocks and we swim in the hidden water.

There were many hidden animals in the jungle below.

There were many many hidden animals in the jungle.

Monkeys would come.

Monkeys would come to the mountains and the trees and we the Drawn People would play with them in the waterfalls.

The Monkeys showed the Drawn People how they exercised and they would swim.

But one day, the Monkeys didn't come.

They had disappeared …

The Drawn People were not the only ones to have noticed that the monkeys had disappeared.

Early morning in the jungle – the jungle below the mountains – the animals were sleeping.

Sabre-toothed Tiger, Snake, Crocodile, Elephant and Giraffe were sleeping …

… waiting for the sun.

When the dawn arrived the animals awoke.

Slowly … stretching … yawning – they woke with the sun.

They rose and readied themselves for breakfast when suddenly – altogether – they sensed danger…

Some prepared to fight.

Some hid.

Some went back to sleep … as the danger swept through the jungle.

Page 1 of 4

The danger passed and a whisper went through the animals.

It was then they too had realised that the monkeys were missing.

The animals held a meeting.

Should they ask for help?

Should they ask the Drawn People for help?

The Drawn People who lived in the Mountains ... who swam with the monkeys ... who hunted the animals in the jungle below?

Snake was worried and wanted to stay.

Elephant was worried and wanted to stay.

Sabre-toothed Tiger was not sure what to do and neither was Giraffe.

It was Crocodile who stepped forward and said 'You are right to be worried over being hunted by The Drawn People, but don't forget – we too have claws. We too have teeth. We too have each other to protect us. We should ask for help.'

With that, the animals went together ... travelling downstream.

Through the mad-grey, white, pink, purple, blue, green, orange, brown and black lands ...

... over the waterfall into the bubbling whirlpool.

Into the water below ...

... where the monkeys used to play and swim.

The Drawn People were already there.

They were looking at the water where they used to swim.

It was disappearing.

Slowly sinking.

Slowly shrinking.

The Drawn People and the Animals looked on as a giant Whale Shark

- a giant, cheeky, nasty, tricky whale shark -

slowly sucked up the water into his HUGE belly.

But it wasn't just water he sucked up.

Whale Shark was sucking up fish. He was sucking up coral. He was sucking up everything that dared to dip its toe into the water.

That's why the monkeys had disappeared. They had been sucked up. They were trapped – inside the belly of the Whale Shark.

The Drawn People had their nets.
The Animals developed a plan.

Using themselves as bait, the Animals distracted the Whale Shark
– the giant, cheeky, nasty, tricky whale shark –
while the Drawn People sneaked ... silently ... still – up to the Whale Shark with their nets.

GOTCHA!!!!!

They caught him. They opened his mouth. They pulled the creatures free.
Swordfish...Fluoro Fish...Lobster...Turtle...Octopus...Seahorse...

...and...

... MONKEY!

There was still a problem though.
Whale Shark was still in the water.
And while Whale Shark was still in the water, they were all in danger.

It was then that Penguin stepped forward.

Penguin was so grateful for being rescued from the HUGE belly of Whale Shark that he decided to let the Drawn People into a secret.

The secret of breathing – underwater...

Penguin supervised as the Drawn People held their breath.

Penguin supervised as the Drawn People practised blowing bubbles. HUGE bubbles.

- giant, cheeky, nasty, tricky bubbles –

These were going to be blown into the belly of the Whale Shark.

Sharpening their spears, the Drawn People dived while the animals kept watch.

Holding their breath the Drawn People approached Whale Shark.

Slowly circling Whale Shark they blew.

BUBBLES.

Bubbles to trap.

Bubbles to pop.

Bubbles to stop Whale Shark.

The bubbles grew –

        BIGGER

           BIGGER

              BIGGER

until Whale Shark's belly was full.

The Drawn People took their spears and …

POP!

Whale Shark exploded.

He exploded with such a force – POP! – that he blew the animals back to the Jungle.

He exploded with such a force – POP! – that he blew the Drawn People back to the Mountains.

He exploded with such a force that he made the Monkeys laugh – POP!

And the Drawn People could swim again.

DEVELOPING CHARACTERS

To help establish the water environment, have two assistants hold the blue material at either end so that individual children can run underneath when it gets wafted into the air.

Alternatively if mobility is an issue, the following rhyme can be used with the material (and vocal energy) mimicking the words:

The sea can be gentle
The sea can be flat
The sea can be calm
As a sleeping cat. [gentle wafting]

THE SEA CAN BE WILD!
THE SEA CAN BE TOUGH!
THE SEA CAN BE LOUD!
THE SEA CAN BE ROUGH! [wildly flapping]

The water mist could also be sprayed over the group during the second stanza.

Note: Spraying with water should only be done with the permission of the group, as some individuals may become distressed at either getting wet or being surprised.

Some people may prefer not to go underneath the material, but will be happy to sit on top instead. If so, ask some of the group to hold the edges of the material while others sit in the centre. Get the people around the edge to gently shake the material to make small waves and play some sea music. Ask those in the centre to try out different swimming movements such as breaststroke, front crawl, floating on the water. If you have sea creature puppets (e.g., fish, dolphins) or objects such as shells, pass these around for the people in the centre to touch and see.

You can also spend some time using the 'water' instruments to explore sounds that can be made at different volumes and speeds. Allow each person to share the sound of their instrument and then add each instrument in turn to create a 'water orchestra'. One person could conduct the orchestra, using their arms or body to indicate to the others whether to play loud or soft, slow or fast.

To finish, the whole group can sit holding the edges of the blue material while the monkeys are placed in the centre. The poem or water orchestra can then be used to guide the actions while the monkeys are tossed around – swimming!

STORY-BUILDING ACTIVITIES

Activity: Sleeping Animals

★ Set up some mats on the floor for the group to use as their animal's home (alternatively you might like to create a special den for the chosen animal).

★ Ask individuals to show you their chosen animal in a frozen pose on their mats.

You might need to spend some time establishing the forest/jungle environment, before everyone settles down in role as an animal. Take the group on an imaginary journey through a forest, crawling through various locations such as muddy swamps, jumping over streams and ducking under branches. Allow different people to lead the expedition (as in the game 'Follow the Leader') making sure the group copy the leader's movements or actions.

Ask questions such as 'What can you see/hear/smell/feel in the forest?' Or, if you have a monkey or parrot puppet, use the puppet in role to lead the group around the forest/jungle. If possible, build a tunnel using tables covered in fabric to add effect to the sense of 'journeying'.

At each location in the forest, allow time for imaginative play e.g., painting mud on faces from the swamp (this could be real mud or water-based face paint), catching fish in the stream or climbing trees.

★ Move on to show how each animal sleeps, what sounds they might make – are they dreaming?

★ Narrate each animal's awakening (you could also do this to music). For example:

> *"Slowly each animal yawned, and stretched and opened its eyes.*
> *They sniffed the air, licked their lips and prepared for breakfast.*
> *As they were eating, they suddenly stopped. Danger was nearby.*
> *Each animal froze ready to run or hide or attack."*

To help guide each person, tap them on the foot or shoulder to encourage them to yawn and awaken. Remind them to stay on their 'acting mat' and encourage the rest of the group by asking the other animals to turn and look (and even copy) while that person repeats a particular activity such as yawning, stretching or holding their frozen animal stance.

★ Ask each animal to freeze again and while frozen, brush past each one with a large piece of material, or alternatively use a feather duster to brush their arms as you narrate, for example:

> *"Finally the danger passed and the frozen animals breathed*
> *a sigh of relief and sat down together."*

★ Finish by asking each animal how they felt and what they thought the danger might be.

Activity: Down The Waterfall

★ Create a 'canoe' using the gym mats (or squares of carpet). Place a volunteer in the canoe, ready to go down the waterfall first. Give everyone else an instrument.

If the time and space are available, you could also create an underwater sensory den. This could involve craft activities such as making silver-foil fish, running through bubbles and activities such as guided movement to music. If available, you could use a fluorescent room.

★ Recite the poem below. When you get to the numbers, guide the rest of the group as they use the various instruments to build the sound and speed until the canoe 'crashes' into the waves at the bottom of the waterfall. The crash can be achieved by the music coming to either a crescendo or stop and the person in the canoe getting sprayed with water (if appropriate) and/or covered up by the blue piece of material.

> Riding faster, riding through
> Here is [name] in their canoe
> Slow at first
> Picking up speed
> They really must be brave indeed.
> 1, 2, 3, 4, 5, 6, 7, 8, 9, 10 … SPLASH !!!!

Activity: Rescuing the Animals

★ To introduce the character of Whale Shark, start making some large 'sucking' sounds as you approach each person while gathering together a variety of sea creatures and/or objects, as if they are being sucked up as you go.

You could also wear a costume such as a large cape or use a prop such as a large bag or basket to help denote the character of Whale Shark and guide the story/ drama with some narration such as:

"I am Whale Shark. I'm very thirsty and I'm drinking up all the water.
Sluuurrrrpppp!"

> **CASE STUDY**
>
> On one occasion during this activity, a number of the children in the group wanted to protect the creatures being sucked up and it developed into a spontaneous game of hide and seek.

Once all the creatures have been collected, Whale Shark (with a full belly) falls asleep!

★ Drop your role and produce the netting. Tell the group that one-by-one they are going to sneak up on the sleeping Whale Shark and capture him in the netting and rescue one of the animals.

★ Resume the role of Whale Shark, asleep on a nearby chair. As each person sneaks up (or is guided to do so by a teaching assistant), they capture Whale Shark by putting the netting over him (TIR).

★ Once you have been caught (in-role), reluctantly give up one of your previously 'sucked up' animals or objects.

★ Individuals can then share what or who they rescued with the rest of the group.

Extensions

★ To extend the 'rescue', various pieces of equipment can be used to create a small obstacle course. Each participant can then be encouraged to make the hazardous journey to rescue the animals, for example, over the hill, through the tunnel, across a spider's web (made of long criss-crossed pieces of elastic). Once they have crossed all the obstacles they will have reached the place where Whale Shark is hiding.

★ Another game can be that every time Whale Shark makes a sound, the rescuers have to freeze (as in 'Grandmother's Footsteps'). This makes the obstacle course even harder to cross.

★ Using a large piece of material (lycra is particularly effective for this activity) allow each group member in turn to experience the feeling of being 'caught' and 'released'. Wrap the lycra around them like a sausage; allow them to move their body within the lycra, and then release them by letting them spin out of the fabric. Find varying ways to use the lyrca to explore the difference between being 'bound' and 'free'. Develop this further by using movement to music with the theme of bound and free. This could be done as individuals, or in pairs or in small groups.

Activity: Blowing Up Whale Shark

★ Invite the group to practise blowing imaginary bubbles by breathing in and holding their breath and blowing out for a count of five. Demonstrate an imaginary bubble by moving your hands wider and wider as you blow them up.

★ Resume your role as Whale Shark and have the group surround you, all holding hands as they repeat the breathing and blowing sequence.

★ As they do this, blow up an actual balloon. When it is full, tie the end, get the group to cover their ears and then burst the balloon. On 'pop', the children can all retreat back to the mats as if being blown back to shore. As a movement activity, encourage the children to retreat back in slow motion as their animals.

For any children who are sound sensitive, you could instead:

– Replace the actual balloon with the group themselves saying 'pop' after a count of five.

– Release the blown-up balloon so it 'fizzles' around the classroom instead of bursting.

– Hold hands in a circle and pretend that the whole circle is the Whale Shark. Start with the circle being as tight together as possible so there's very little space in the middle. Slowly begin to move outwards until everyone's arms are fully stretched.

Count down '3, 2, 1...' and then all shout 'Pop!' letting go of hands and falling to the floor. Repeat the exercise using a parachute, where everyone is hidden underneath the parachute, holding the edges down behind their backs. As you count down and shout 'Pop!' let the parachute fall to the floor in the middle.

★ End the workshop by repeating the activity of swimming with the monkeys (see 'Developing Characters', p. 135).

FURTHER DEVELOPMENT

If you have a moderately verbal group, set up a discussion or debate about how Whale Shark felt about being captured and exploded. Ask someone to volunteer to be in-role as Whale Shark, while the others take on the role of the rescued creatures. Set up a debate about whether or not Whale Shark should have been exploded and allow everyone to voice their opinion.

Story Drama for People with Complex Disabilities

Blue Fish

ORIGINAL SETTING

The story of Blue Fish was developed during a six-week residency in a Special Educational Needs primary school, working with pupils aged 10 to 12 years who had severe and complex learning disabilities and some physical impairment.

All pupils were able to make simple choices, using eye-points or reaching for a particular symbol or object they wished to use. Most were learning to create simple sentences using various electronic communication devices.

PREPARATION

These weekly workshops lasted between 45 minutes and an hour in the group's classroom after their regular morning greetings. Each workshop involved eight pupils, one classroom teacher and four support workers. All pupils and staff were seated in a circle on either chairs, squares of carpet or beanbags.

When working with those with complex learning disabilities it is advisable to arrange planning visits prior to your first official workshop.

Such visits will help you to:

★ Liaise with the classroom teacher regarding the content of the workshops and if appropriate establish individual learning outcomes for each pupil.

★ Decide on the most productive space to use; it may be better to keep the group in their regular classroom space, as moving them could waste time and disrupt the involvement of certain members of the group.

★ Evaluate how each group member communicates.

★ Allow time for the class to get used to the routine of you being there.

★ Introduce and experiment with some of the drama activities you will use during the workshops.

AIMS

As well as individual targets, the overall aim of this project was to give the group the opportunity to devise and enact their own story.

CASE STUDY

As the class had already been exploring natural elements, it was decided to expand on this theme looking at both the ocean and the earth, and the creatures that live in both environments.

The weekly workshops were designed to help them explore these worlds and the characters, while discovering and developing individual voices. In addition, it was important to promote and encourage their ownership of the work produced.

In your own setting, the project could culminate in a class assembly showcasing some of the workshop activities or the presentation of a book in which each pupil's story is recorded.

Each week revisit the same workshop to help reinforce the drama activities introduced, however, aim to change the group's focus to different characters, allowing different pupils to take the lead.

If you do intend to create a book or written record of the project, ensure you allow for the time it will take to honour each pupil's voice in the stories created. You could develop a routine of recording the workshop sessions, allowing you to directly scribe the story as it develops. Be aware though – as a writer or scriber – of finding a balance between 'shaping' the work produced and wanting to rewrite it to make it 'better'!

Evaluation

Just as planning and preparation are important to the success of the workshop, so is having time to reflect on the project once it is completed.

Feedback to the class teacher can help to monitor how well a pupil's individual contributions have influenced and been incorporated into the work, or the degree to which they were able to fully participate in the workshops without incident. Observations such as this can help in the development of any future work.

THE STORY STRUCTURE

Props & Materials

You will need:

★ Blue card with a picture of the sea

★ Music to represent the sea (suggestion: Tchaikovsky's lake scene from *Swan Lake*)

★ Brown card with a picture of the earth

★ Music to represent the earth (suggestion: Mozart's *Rondo* from 'Horn Concerto No.4')

★ Salt-water spray bottle

★ A container filled with flour

★ A collection of stuffed animals/creatures (or picture representations) for both the sea and the earth

Sample Scripts

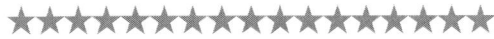

★★★★★★★★★★★★★★★★★★★★★

THE STORY OF BLUE FISH

Once upon a time, under the sea, there lived a Blue Fish who had a strange habit of swimming upside down.

'I like swimming upside down!', he would say, as he happily saw the world from this strange angle.

Other sea creatures wondered why he swam upside down and thought he might need help learning how to swim the right way up, but all Blue Fish ever said to them was,

'I like swimming upside down!'

One day, as he was swimming upside down, he saw the King of the World arrive. Blue Fish was so excited that he rushed to get the King's crown and red cape to give to him.

There was much fanfare as the other animals lined up to greet the King. They bowed low as Blue Fish solemnly presented the King with his crown and delicately placed the red cape about his shoulders.

After the official greeting, the King turned to Blue Fish.

'Hello Blue Fish. I have come to warn you and all the creatures who live under the sea that a storm is coming.'

The other creatures were worried, but Blue Fish knew what to do. He showed them all how to escape the rising waters and as the storm approached each creature swam low, so low, underneath the swelling waves and were safe.

Once the storm had passed, Blue Fish jumped for joy, high among the now still waves, diving and swimming as he always did … upside down!

THE STORY OF THE CRAB & THE CROCODILE

Once upon a time under the sea there lived a mean old Crocodile who snapped at anybody who came near him.

He would amuse himself by pretending to be asleep while other sea creatures would sneak up as close as they dared. Crocodile would then scare them away by roaring and snapping.

One day, as he was playing this game, Crab came along and crept closer than anyone ever had crept before and poked out her tongue. Crocodile was so surprised that he almost forgot to roar and snap, but when he realised what this little Crab had done, he got so angry he roared louder than he had ever roared before.

But nothing happened. Crab didn't run away. Instead, she went and got all the other creatures that Crocodile used to roar and snap at and showed them what had happened. She actually poked her tongue out at Crocodile again! This confused Crocodile and made him even angrier. Just as he was about to do something, a fanfare was heard.

The King of the World was coming. The King turned to Crocodile.
'Hello Crocodile. Have you heard? A storm is coming.'

Crocodile suddenly forgot how angry he was and watched while the King showed the other creatures how to escape the rising water.

Once the storm had passed, Crocodile didn't see Crab again.
'She must have learned her lesson!' he thought.

After the storm, Crab didn't see Crocodile again.
'He must have learned his lesson!' she thought.

HANDOUT 18

SEAHORSE & LOBSTER

Deep down under the sea there lived a Seahorse who was sad because his friend the Lobster was away. Other sea creatures tried to cheer him up but whenever they asked Seahorse if he was feeling better, all he would say was …

'No!'

Suddenly, news reached him of a special visitor under the sea. It was the King of the World. Despite news of the storm, Seahorse smiled at the thought of meeting someone so important and watched as the King of the World showed him how to escape the rising water.

Once the storm had passed, Seahorse was so happy to see his friend the Lobster swimming high among the waves that he swam over to him and together they played their favourite game!

★ A King's cape and crown

★ Music for an earthquake (suggestion: Greig's *In The Hall Of The Mountain King*)

★ Music for a storm (suggestion: Vivaldi's *Summer* from 'The Four Seasons')

★ A fanfare for the King's entrance

★ A written royal proclamation/warning, e.g., a scroll

★ Parachute material

★ Percussion instruments (optional)

STORY-BUILDING ACTIVITIES

Activity: Establish a Location

★ Place both the brown earth card and blue sea card in the middle of the circle.

★ After greeting each member of the group, choose someone to decide for the group where they would like to play that day.

★ Once chosen, sing the following song using either a salt-water spray or tub of flour to enhance the sensory experience of their choice.

Note: When using these, ensure that each person is comfortable being sprayed with water or sprinkled with the earth. For those that are more sensitive, options can include lightly touching their lips for them to taste the salt or dabbing the water on their hands for them to lick off. The tub of flour can either be sprinkled lightly over them or they can be encouraged to dip their hands in to feel the texture. You might also want to experiment with different textures such as brown sugar, porridge oats, sand or soil.

> Playing in the sea/earth
> Playing in the sea/earth
> Look at [name of pupil]
> Look at [name of pupil]
> Playing in the sea/earth
> (*Sung to the tune of 'Knees Up Mother Brown'*)

CASE STUDY

In one class, a pupil had an issue with cleanliness and became quite alarmed at the thought of getting dirty. After three sessions of watching others get grubby playing in the earth he finally put his hands into the tub of flour and without warning threw it all over me, I laughed and repeated his action by throwing even more flour over my head. Suddenly he copied my action by throwing flour all over himself! This developed into a movement activity with everyone stamping feet, clapping hands and shaking their heads and, for that day at least, he didn't mind getting grubby. However, from then on, every other child insisted on covering me in flour!

Activity: Choosing Characters

★ Place a selection of stuffed animals/creatures (or picture representations) associated with either the sea or the earth in the centre of the circle. Now invite the group to choose which animal they would like to be.

★ Once chosen, say the following rhyme.

> Hey, hey can it be.
> Who's this saying hi to me?
> [character] … [character]
> Hello [character]
> It's time to play … in the [environment].

This rhyme is also an ideal way to say goodbye to each character at the end of the drama workshop.

CASE STUDY

I was concerned that there might be an initial conflict with two pupils wanting the same creature, however, this never occurred (although if it had it would have been the ideal opportunity to encourage sharing or to explore the story/drama of this conflict). In fact, the pupils became so attached to their characters that the moment the environment for the day was chosen they would all be eager to be reunited with their animals, one pupil eventually took the role upon himself of distributing the various characters to their respective owners.

Activity: Character Movements & Sounds

★ Play the piece of music chosen to represent either the sea or the earth so the group can demonstrate how their character might move. Prompt with simple choices such as: do they move fast or slowly? Are they big or small?

★ Further character developments can include questions such as how is your character feeling (happy or sad)? Is your character mean or friendly?

★ Introduce these character choices to the rest of the group and get them to either copy or react to them.

CASE STUDY

From this basic activity, any drama can develop. We had the character of crocodile who liked scaring and snapping at the other animals, who would run away from him. This game soon developed into the story of crab *not* running away from crocodile and with crab teaching the other characters how to stand up to crocodile.

During another session, one pupil (lobster) was away, which affected the participation and behaviour of another (seahorse). We managed to include his sadness into that week's workshop and the following week when lobster returned we recapped his story and developed it further.

CASE STUDY

As groups become more familiar and you start to better understand individual communication choices, you can be more adventurous and confident with character interactions. In one group there was a boy with autism and very limited speech. He would occasionally (if prompted) point to the pupil he wanted the group to sing to next, but often that would be the extent of his involvement in the entire workshop. While exploring the characters of the earth, he chose to be monkey. I developed the game 'Monkey Tickle', in which he would point to a pupil who would then be tickled by the 'mischievous' monkey for a count of ten (I would tickle the person with a feather duster). Some of the other pupils enjoyed the tickling sessions, some didn't, but at least monkey was now engaged further within the workshop and it provided a wonderful narrative for his developing story.

Activity: The King's Warning

★ Show the King's crown and cape to the group.

★ Practise staging a royal entrance complete with a fanfare and bowing as the King approaches and greets each animal or creature. This could initially be done by you demonstrating the role of the King before repeating with one (or a number) of the group taking over the role themselves.

★ The King gives a warning that either a storm or an earthquake is coming (depending on which environment you have been playing in that day). This could be done verbally or in the form of a written proclamation that is then read and shown to the group.

★ Use the parachute material and music to help create either the storm or the earthquake.

For the storm, have two assistants hold either end of the parachute, wafting it high in the air as individual participants (with their chosen characters) escape underneath from one side to the other. Water can also be sprayed to help add to the effect.

For the earthquake, have the group hold the edges of the parachute as each of the stuffed animal characters is placed on top of the material and bounced. If picture representations are being used instead, then try placing a foam ball or other soft object in the centre of the parachute for the group to bounce around. Some group members might also like to sit underneath the material while the earthquake is taking place. Percussion instruments such as drums and shakers can also be introduced for the group to use while sitting underneath the material.

CASE STUDY

One pupil took on the role of the 'King of the World' for himself. One day, I tried to introduce some drama for him by declaring that we couldn't find his crown, hoping that this would develop into a unique storyline with the other characters helping to look for it. However, the King, unperturbed by my announcement, promptly improvised a crown with some paper and proceeded with his royal duties. Yet another reminder that no matter what my intentions, I still had to honour the story being created!

FURTHER DEVELOPMENT

Further story developments could include exploring each character's daily routines, for example, what they eat, how old they are, do they go to school or work and developing their individual family life. For group members with severe and complex disabilities, understanding and separating their own life from that of their character can sometimes be hard to achieve. However, this extension can help keep those with more moderate learning disabilities engaged if you are working with a mixed group.

Another drama development for groups with moderate learning disabilities could include the introduction of a dilemma such as: 'The King of the World has lost his power and therefore can't predict any more storms or earthquakes'. The characters could discuss why the King has lost his power and prepare for a quest to different environments to look for the lost power. This could lead to an exploration of how each character would be able to travel in each environment, exploring the problems of a fish needing to travel above ground.

Adolescent Groups with Autism Spectrum Disorders

AZ & the McPuppets

ORIGINAL SETTING

The following workshop was developed as part of a seven-week school residency working with a small group of boys with ASD aged 15 to 17 years. These boys had little drama experience, limited communication skills and many were extremely sound sensitive. They could all make choices, provided these were not over-complicated and clear instruction was both given and repeated. Their understanding of the world was 'in the moment' and they had difficulty with any references to the past or using their imagination to pretend they were elsewhere.

BSL (British Sign Language) and Makaton signs and symbols were used to aid communication and most of the boys enjoyed drawing and creating pictures. Photographic displays were also prevalent in the classroom to help provide a reference of daily activities and past experiences.

The group would have up to an hour-and-a-half contact time per week in which to create individual stories that would then be staged in an assembly presentation. The first hour of each workshop was for practical drama activities with the last half hour spent helping the boys to fill in worksheets, draw character pictures or create their puppets.

Each session was initially planned for the small carpeted area of the classroom to minimise distress to the participants. However, as the boys became more used to the scheduled sessions, the school drama studio was also used and the boys were comfortable moving to this new location provided enough notice was given.

PREPARATION

Prior to the first official workshop, try to arrange some pre-visits. These visits will provide an opportunity to consult with the class teacher on possible themes and discuss how the project could enhance any topics currently being studied. It will also give the group the chance to meet and get comfortable with you as a visiting practitioner.

In addition to discussions with the class teacher, the aim of the pre-visits can be to observe and assess the following:

★ How the teacher works with individuals.

★ How individual pupils communicate and make choices.

★ How you could adapt or manipulate the space to be used for the workshops.

Other pre-visits can then allow you to run a number of simple drama activities, increasing your understanding of how each pupil communicates and makes choices.

These exercises can also highlight other adjustments that may need to be made, for example:

★ Ensuring that your instructions are not too complex.

★ Monitoring the tone and volume of your voice.

After the pre-visits, you may be aware of a variety of other challenges which will need to be considered prior to the first workshop. For example:

★ Is there enough time for the group to develop and build belief in the created world and its characters, taking into account the time needed for weekly repetition and re-capping?

★ Can the group explore drama from a collective problem-solving perspective?

★ What are the individual communication needs and how can they be utilised to make choices?

★ What is each student's level of literacy?

★ Will you have time to find a balance between producing an assembly presentation and allowing the group time to develop and explore their stories?

AIMS

The initial aim for this group was to develop characters that were not human, such as objects, animals, elements or creatures. There were two reasons for this. First, to see how far the young people with complex ASD could comprehend, commit to and develop abstract characters. Secondly, by using abstract figures we hoped to provide a safety net for the participants, allowing human emotions and dilemmas to be explored while preventing any possible identifying connections or embarrassments between them. The stories created were written into script format, while the group recorded their experiences in the form of worksheets, photographs and sound recordings.

CASE STUDY

As the boys had recently had a day trip to London that included lunch at a well-known fast-food restaurant, we decided to use this experience as the basis for their story. Of course, focusing on the theme of fast food may not be appropriate for all groups and it could be that you wish to adapt the following workshop in order to promote healthier eating if this is important in your setting.

The character of 'AZ' was inspired by the London A-Z guide book, while the practical nature of creating puppet characters from fast-food containers became an extremely useful tool as it:

★ Helped create ownership of their developing stories.

★ Allowed the boys to share in a collective dramatic experience.

★ Aided in the distinction between themselves and their characters.

Keep in mind that people with autism may have difficulty distinguishing between their own emotions and those of the characters. Despite reservations about whether this was possible to achieve, the teachers commented that the boys' personalities were clearly apparent in the devised stories and it was obvious that they had benefited from the experience.

When judging the success of the project, the following points should be taken into consideration:

★ Were the group able to remember and relate to the work produced?

★ Was the work followed up through the week by the teachers or referred to by the group?

★ Did the group have ownership of the work? That is, did it provide a vehicle for their individual artistic voices?

THE STORY STRUCTURE

Props & Materials

You will need:

★ A selection of clothes and costume items

★ A selection of emotion picture cards showing happy, sad, angry, faces (optional)

★ The covers of a guidebook

★ A selection of 'food' cards (such as pictures of baked beans, cakes, hamburgers, cereal). (You will need two of each food item, with one 'odd one out'.)

★ An apron

★ A tablecloth, cutlery, salt & pepper shakers etc

★ A tray

★ A selection of clean fast-food containers, e.g., clam-shell style boxes, drinks containers

★ A selection of environment picture cards e.g., rubbish bin, refrigerator, food tray, kitchen, a table and a chair

★ Water-based marker pens

★ A collection of craft materials such as wool, glue, stick-on eyes

★ A camera (ensure you have appropriate permission to take photographs)

★ Copies of the worksheets or blank paper

Sample Script– AZ & the McPuppets

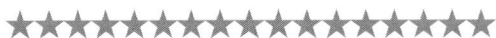

★★★★★★★★★★★★★★★★★★

The following is an amalgamation of the individual stories developed. In addition to the scripts, the completed book (which was presented to the group at the end of the project) also contained the worksheets used and photographs of the group dressed as 'AZ' and holding their McPuppets.

SCENE 1 – Meeting AZ

Narrator:	This is AZ.
	AZ appears, dressed in green shirt, sunglasses, tartan hat and fluffy ears. He is carrying a deflated balloon.
Narrator:	Today AZ is feeling rather sad for a lot of different reasons. First …
AZ:	My balloon burst.
Narrator:	Second …
AZ:	Somebody hit me!
Narrator:	… and third …
AZ:	I've got spots all over my face – chicken pox!
Narrator:	… but despite all these things, AZ was putting on a brave face.
AZ:	*(putting on his brave face)* I don't feel sad.
Narrator:	In fact, to cheer himself up, he decided to go and treat himself at the shop to his all-time favourite food.
AZ:	Fish & Chips!
Narrator:	When AZ got to the shop, it was so busy that he was asked if he could help out. AZ loved putting on the shopkeeper's uniform and was happy to help behind the counter with all the customers.

Unfortunately, by the time he finished serving, there was no food left.

Shop Keeper: All gone.

Narrator: This only made AZ sad again.

AZ: Boo-Hoo.

Narrator: Until the shopkeeper suggested that he go to a local restaurant.

SCENE 2 – The Restaurant

Narrator: On the other side of town, living quite happily inside the restaurant was a chicken sandwich.

Chicken Sandwich: Yes!

Narrator: Chicken Sandwich was old, but very happy and spent his days sitting on a food tray by the window.

Chicken Sandwich: Yes!

Narrator: Occasionally he would get glimpses of his friend Chicken Roll as the door to the kitchen swung open and smells from his old environment wafted through the restaurant.

                 CHICKEN SANDWICH breathes in deeply and sighs as he waves to CHICKEN ROLL.

Narrator: The reason Chicken Sandwich had lasted so long on his food tray was due to a game he used to play on anyone who tried to eat him. He would keep very still and very quiet until someone came up close and then in a big loud voice he would scare them by saying …

Chicken Sandwich: Yes! Yes! Yes! Yes!

Narrator: … and making chomping movements with his mouth towards their nose.

CHICKEN SANDWICH demonstrates this to the audience.

Narrator: Only when someone asked politely would he allow them to take a bite, but usually they just ran away, holding their noses and feeling lucky that they themselves hadn't been eaten!

Chicken Sandwich: Yes! Yes! Yes! Yes!

Narrator: One day, while Chicken Sandwich was sitting on his food tray, AZ appeared in the restaurant singing ...

AZ: Going to the restaurant (Going to the restaurant)
And what shall I eat? (And what shall I eat?)
[name of pupil] going to have ... (repeated)
[type of food] (repeated)

SCENE 3 – Cleaning Up

Narrator: When AZ arrived at the restaurant, he couldn't believe his eyes. It was filthy. There was an old drink container under the chair, an over-flowing rubbish bin outside the door, strange smells wafting in from the kitchen and sitting by the window on a food tray was an old chicken sandwich.

Narrator: This would not do. AZ decided to clean up. He found a cloth and started to clean the windows.

AZ starts his window-cleaning action.

Narrator: This cleaning started to worry Chicken Sandwich.

Chicken Sandwich: Yes!

Narrator: So he decided to run away and hide. At first he ran and hid under a chair with Orange Squash, but AZ found them.

AZ: Yes!

Narrator: Then he decided to run away and hide in the kitchen.

Chicken Sandwich: Yes!

Narrator:	He took Orange Squash with him, but AZ found them there too.
AZ:	Yes!
Narrator:	Finally Chicken Sandwich had the perfect idea for a hiding place. He took Orange Squash with him and they both ran outside and hid in the rubbish bin with Old Hamburger.
Chicken Sandwich:	Yes!
Narrator:	Unfortunately, the rubbish bin was exactly where AZ wanted them to go, and now, they were stuck!
AZ:	Yes!
Narrator:	Chicken Sandwich didn't want to stay in the rubbish bin. He liked his space on the food tray.
Chicken Sandwich:	Yes!
Narrator:	But just as he began to feel sad at the thought of not being able to look out of the window again, his old friend Chicken Roll came to the rescue. He had cleverly crept behind AZ when he wasn't looking, and lifted the lid off the rubbish bin. Chicken Sandwich was free.
Chicken Sandwich:	Yes!
Narrator:	He was about to thank his friend for rescuing him, but Chicken Roll was already making his way back into the restaurant, talking about a plan to stop AZ from cleaning up once and for all. Chicken Sandwich didn't mind him going as he happily made his way back into the restaurant, where he found his food tray waiting for him and the world passing by outside the window.
Chicken Sandwich:	Yes!
Narrator:	Although he did wonder about AZ and his cleaning cloth. Would they ever come back again … ?

SCENE 4 – The Vacuum Cleaner

Narrator: While AZ was making his way back into the restaurant, Chicken Roll was hatching a plan.

Chicken Roll: Yes!

Narrator: The restaurant had a faulty vacuum cleaner. Anyone trying to use it had to be very careful that the setting was switched to 'SLOW'. Otherwise the 'FAST' setting would spin them around and wrap them up in the power cord. Chicken Roll's plan was to fiddle with the switch so that it would only be on 'FAST'. He then placed the vacuum cleaner by the open kitchen door.

Chicken Roll: Yes!

Narrator: Just as he had made the adjustments and hidden out of sight, AZ came out of the kitchen. He was looking puzzled. Then he spotted the vacuum cleaner.

AZ demonstrates the following action sequence.

Narrator: AZ plugged in the vacuum cleaner. He positioned himself close to the kitchen door and held the hose in front of him.

AZ: Ready!

Narrator: He turned the power switch ON.

AZ: *(spinning wildly out the door)* Aaaahh!!

Narrator: The vacuum cleaner took control of AZ and he spun round and round the kitchen.

Sounds of broken crockery and glasses smashing are heard off-stage.

Narrator: Then suddenly, all was quiet.

The noise stops.

Narrator: Chicken Roll crept out of his hiding place and back into the kitchen. There was no sign of AZ or the vacuum cleaner and he hoped that was the last time anyone would try to tidy up his lovely restaurant.

Page 5 of 5

You could use the following call and response rhyme to introduce and end each session. Spend a little time recapping the previous week's drama (either through narration, role-play or repeating moments that were particularly successful) before moving forward.

We're gonna make a play
With people here today
Who do we have?
Let's say Hi!
Hi [name of participant]
It's time to start!

We all made a play
With people here today
Who did we have?
Let's say Bye!
Bye [name of participant]
I'll see you soon.

STORY-BUILDING ACTIVITIES

Activity: *Creating the character of 'AZ'*

★ Place a collection of clothes and costume items on the floor in themed groups, for example a pile of shirts, a selection of glasses, hats and wigs, trousers etc.

★ Ask the group to decide on the following:

  – Which pair of glasses does he wear (sunglasses/spectacles)?

  – Does he wear a hat or a wig?

  – Which shirt does he wear?

  – Does AZ walk on two or four legs?

  – Does he speak English?

★ Once the costume has been chosen, have individuals dress up in the clothes (or, as they make each decision, put the costume on yourself).

★ Take photographs of each member of the group wearing the costume of AZ.

If group members are either afraid or embarrassed to dress up, you could demonstrate the character and greet each person. You may find that most of the group are then eager to dress up and 'play' as the character of AZ, while others may remain quite nervous and even run away from the character. Others still may just want to watch the action from the corner of the room. However, over time you should find that everyone will eventually want to participate in some way.

Activity: Exploring Emotions

★ While individuals are wearing the costume you might like to ask AZ how is he feeling (use questions such as, 'Is AZ feeling sad or happy?'). Ask the group to show how AZ would stand if he was feeling a particular emotion, encouraging them to also try displaying this emotion on their faces. Other questions could include:

  – Do you like your clothes?

  – Do you have any family?

  – Do you have any hobbies?

★ To help groups with more complex disabilities make emotional choices for their characters, use the emotion cards (happy, sad, angry) for them to choose from. Individually or collectively the group can:

  – Look at the face. Copy the face. Decide on the emotion.

  – Suggest what you might say or do if you were feeling that emotion.

  – Rehearse an interaction (if possible).

Note: If participants have more complex ASD, ensure you provide definite choices of emotions from which to choose answers. Be aware of the effects of some images, for instance the emotion card for angry could raise issues with regards to behaviour. Some of the group could become over-excited and the actions associated with certain emotions (such as a fist smacking into a hand to show anger) can sometimes be discouraged within schools. Try to balance expressions of emotion in the workshop with the work on emotions and managing feelings already being carried out by the school.

Many groups with ASD may have issues around the differences between 'stage play' and 'real life' expressions of emotion. You may well find that despite asking the questions in the third person, the responses you receive will be in the first person. However, this can help you ascertain how each person is feeling that day.

★ End the session by having the group draw a picture of AZ (Handout 20). If possible get them to add a speech bubble with some further character information, such as 'My name is AZ and I am feeling [chosen emotion].' Or 'My name is AZ and I like [hobby].' (Handout 21).

Activity: The Special Handshake

★ Go up to each participant, shake their hand and say 'hello'.

★ Ask the group to greet each other.

★ Bring out the costume choices for AZ.

Note: If working over a number of sessions, you might like to recap by looking at the pictures drawn of AZ and revisit the costume and character choices from the first activity 'Creating the character of AZ'.

★ Ask the group to develop a special handshake and greeting for AZ. If necessary ask them to respond 'yes' or 'no' to the choices you provide. For example:

– Does AZ smile when he meets someone?

– Does he shake their hand?

– Is it different from the way *we* shake hands?

– Can you show me how it's different?

★ Have someone (or yourself) dress up as AZ and get them to greet the other participants. Remind them to use the special handshake and greeting.

Activity: The Empty Guidebook

★ Dressed in the chosen costume, take on the role of AZ and ask the group to look at your face and body to see if they can guess how AZ might be feeling (in this case sad).

★ Take off the costume and discuss possible reasons for the sadness.

★ Show the group the guidebook covers, noting that it has no pages.

★ Resume the role, and reveal that AZ is sad as he has lost all the pages of his guidebook. Ask the group if they will help you create pages for your guidebook.

The group might want to know how the pages got lost. For example, were they blown away in the wind? Did the dog eat them? You might like to then spend time recreating the moments when AZ lost the pages from his guidebook. This could be done with still images or short improvisations (and might even lead to a whole new story).

★ Tell the group that the first place AZ needs to find is somewhere he can get food because he is hungry.

★ Ask the group to draw pictures of their favourite food and/or restaurant for AZ's guidebook.

Activity: The Shopkeeper

★ Set up a shop environment, by laying one of each of the food cards on a table.

★ Give a selection of the matching food card pairs to the group.

★ In-role as the shopkeeper (wearing the apron), welcome participants to your shop. Ask them what they would like to buy and ask individuals (in-role as customers) to match their food cards to the corresponding ones on the shop table.

If you would like to add another layer to this activity for higher-ability groups, each food card could also be marked with a price. Group members will then have to produce the correct play money to pay for each item.

Activity: AZ at the Shop

★ To introduce the idea of AZ into the shop, either take on the role of the shopkeeper and ask someone in the group dress as AZ, or cast one of the group as the shopkeeper and take on the role of AZ yourself. Encourage the group to show AZ what they have already learned about how to get food from the shop, i.e., matching the various food cards.

★ Eventually take on the role of AZ yourself, however, this time you enter the shop with the odd-one-out food card (the one without a pair). Acting sad, ask the group what you should do next. Where can AZ go to get food?

★ Ask each person to choose their favourite food and share these with the group using the following call and response chant:

Going to the restaurant (Going to the restaurant)
And what shall I eat? (And what shall I eat?)
[name of pupil] going to have … (repeated)
[type of food] (repeated)

Note: This chant could be adapted to any environment or place. For example, going to the park and what shall we play?

Activity: Entering the Restaurant

★ Set up the room as a restaurant with the tablecloth, cutlery and salt and pepper props. You could use a costume item to help denote the character of a waiter and the group could even create menus with their favourite recipes on them.

★ Once the group has settled into their seats, give them the following information (this can be done in-role as the waiter): 'This restaurant is not like any other restaurant. The food here talks.'

★ Place the various fast-food containers on the tray and encourage individuals to slowly approach and make their selection. As each does, startle them by having the food container respond in a way appropriate to each individual.

Note: Startle the group gently as people with ASD can become genuinely frightened. The interaction should be fun and engrossing rather than distressing.

You could encourage each person to approach and order their food. When they lean close to take their choice, surprise them with the food box saying either 'No, No, No' or 'Yes, Yes, Yes'. You could then reverse the roles, asking them to scare you with their food containers when you ask to share some food.

Activity: Making Puppets

★ Using the food containers as a mouth, the group can create puppets by sticking on eyes, creating a tongue and adding hair.

★ To aid in the development of their characters, ask questions such as 'Is your puppet old or young?' and, if appropriate, 'How does he/she/it feel?'

★ Encourage them to add sound to their newly created puppets. These could be a repetition of dialogue spoken in the restaurant scene or might be something completely new.

★ Take a photograph of each participant holding their puppet or ask them to draw a picture of their puppet character. (Handout 22)

★ Ask everyone to name their puppet.

Activity: The McPuppet Locations

★ Place five environment picture cards around the room where they can be easily seen. If possible, you could place them on corresponding items or locations within the space, e.g., if the room has a refrigerator or kitchen area for example.

★ Call out different locations in random order and get the group (with their puppets) to congregate at that particular place. You could add an action and/or sound to each space, for example, when they reach the refrigerator they 'shiver' or for 'under a chair' they bob down.

★ Once the group have explored the various locations, ask them to choose where their puppet lives within the restaurant and to place their puppet on that particular card. For example, do they live:

- In the rubbish bin

- In the refrigerator

- On a food tray

- In the kitchen

- Under a chair

Activity: AZ The Cleaner

★ Through narration, introduce the character of AZ into the restaurant. For example, 'AZ has a new job as a cleaner, but doesn't know how to clean. Can you help him?' Or 'AZ noticed how messy the restaurant was and decided to clean it up.'

★ Get suggestions from the group for different ways and means of cleaning such as wiping windows, dusting, using a mop or vacuuming.

★ Explore the movements and sounds for each of these cleaning activities.

★ In role as AZ, get each member of the group to show you how to clean using the different methods.

CASE STUDY

Our vacuum cleaner developed three settings, slow, fast and very, very fast. Not only did this development prove invaluable for the story, it was also the first time that the group was prepared to accept an 'imaginary' object, even noting where the pretend switch was to turn it on and off.

★ Using the location cards, re-introduce each character's chosen location and place them in those positions around the space.

★ In-role, give the group the bad news that 'AZ has been told to clean you all up and throw you all away'.

★ Have some fun as AZ by cleaning up around the characters. Introduce a 'safe' rule, for example if AZ makes his way to the kitchen, anyone hiding there must freeze and they will be safe.

★ End the session by dropping role and asking the group:

  – Did the characters want to be cleaned up and thrown away?

  – What are we going to do to stop AZ from cleaning?

FURTHER DEVELOPMENT

A restaurant is only one possible location. AZ could visit different environments and interact with characters specific to that location, for example, going to the supermarket and meeting a tin can or to the museum and meeting a dinosaur.

Although the aim of the project was for pupils to devise their own short play for a school assembly, the script developed could be given to another group to rehearse and perform back to the initial 'playwrights'.

Worksheet 1

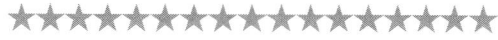

Name: _____

This is AZ.

Worksheet 2

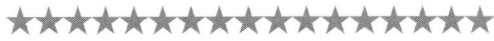

Name: _____

AZ is feeling _____

AZ likes _____

_____

_____

Worksheet 3

Name: ....

This is my puppet character

Its name is ....

It likes to ....

....

Worksheet 4

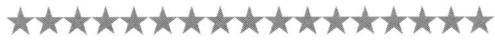

Name: _____

HANDOUT 23

My puppet is feeling _____

This is what it said _____

_____

_____

PART III

Using Existing Stories as a Starter

INTRODUCTION

The focus of this book has so far been on developing original stories through various play activities and drama processes. Yet there could be occasions when the use of an existing story is the best place to start. As already demonstrated in 'Clue Bags', a workshop can help compliment an established story. If you are new to facilitating storytelling or drama work, then using an existing story can also offer you more of a safety net when first working with a group.

There are infinite ways of using an existing story to begin a creative session. For example, if looking at the fairytale 'Cinderella', why not start the workshop from the 'happily ever after' part of the story? Pose questions to the group such as: Is Cinderella truly happy to be married? Does she stay in touch with her family? How does she spend her day now? What happened to the ugly sisters? Who did the fairy godmother help next? This could lead into a re-enactment, quests, still images or movement and sound activities, using many of the workshop structures already outlined. Alternatively, hearing a traditional tale can simply prompt people into telling stories themselves, relating what they've heard to their own life and recalling experiences.

Stories are there to be adapted and explored in any way that your group finds interesting, so keep your mind open to where the group wants to take them. Using existing stories is not simply about re-enactments or retellings, but is a chance to inspire the group and help them access the themes and meanings within each unique tale.

Working in Mixed Inclusive Settings

Dream Catchers (*The BFG*)

ORIGINAL SETTING

'Dream Catchers' was a ten-week collaborative project with an inclusive group of primary-age children from three schools (one mainstream and two SEN schools) using the 'Dream Catcher' elements of Roald Dahl's *The BFG* (Big Friendly Giant) as its focus. The aim was to offer the children a chance to explore the idea of dreams through a series of weekly drama workshops, culminating in a devised performance to be shared with friends and family. Sometimes the workshops involved working with the classes separately in their own settings, whilst some sessions were conducted collaboratively, bringing the groups together.

The idea of using *The BFG* as a starting point for creative drama work was inspiring, both for the facilitators and the children. They were initially asked to think about their own dreams before exploring a number of questions in relation to the story: How might you catch a dream? What happens if a dream is trapped in a jar? What sounds do dreams make? What is the difference between a dream and a nightmare? Most of the children involved in the project were familiar with the story, which meant that we had their interest from the outset. We were also given free rein to explore the theme of dreams however we wished, using a combination of music and drama in order to devise the performance piece.

Using a piece of classic children's literature such as this for creative drama and story-making work can be valuable on many levels. It can enhance the children's understanding and insight into the themes of the book, expanding their literacy skills within the classroom. It can also offer groups of children with particular needs an opportunity to access the story according to their preferred learning style. Many classic children's stories such as this are incredibly rich and touch on universal themes about the human condition. By exploring such themes in a drama context, you are offering your groups the chance to embody and enact these concepts connecting with the story on a deeper level.

The following workshop is an example of how you could explore the story of *The BFG* with any group. You will see that these activities relate directly to the original story, while in the 'Further Development' section you will find examples of how you might simply use the theme of dreams as a starting point for creative work with any age group. If working with the original story directly, you may find it useful to begin a session by reading a relevant section of the book aloud, perhaps using background music to enhance the atmosphere.

THE WORKSHOP

Props & Materials

You will need:

★ Some 'Dream Jars', clear plastic jars or tubs holding a variety of interesting materials such as coloured feathers, curled-up colourful pipe cleaners, glitter, slime

★ A range of colourful ribbons or sparkling pieces of tinsel

★ A range of percussion instruments

★ Pots of bubbles

★ Classical music of various styles to suggest different dream 'types'

★ A container/bowl/bucket to use to mix a 'dream potion'

Activity: Big & Little

★ As a warm-up game, invite the group to explore being big and little to music.

★ Now ask everyone to find a space in the room facing you. You will need a large, clear space for this exercise.

★ With the group, develop an action which can be done on the spot, each with a sound, for each of the following instructions:

  – As BIG as a giant.

  – As SMALL a child.

  – As WIDE as a cave.

  – As FREE as a dream.

★ Once the group have learned the action and sound for each instruction, call them out at random so that the group don't know what is coming next. Try it really fast and see if they can keep up. You can repeat the same instruction twice in a row, for example: *'As big as a giant! As wide as a cave! As free as a dream! As free as a dream! As big as a giant! As small a child! As big as a giant!'*

★ Feel free to add any other instructions that fit with a theme or character from the story.

Activity: BFG Footsteps

★ This game is yet another example of how to use an adaptation of the classic game 'Grandmother's Footsteps' to help engage the group quickly while building tension and belief in the imagined world.

★ The facilitator can be in-role as the BFG (using your physicality and voice to appear big) and the children have to creep up on you across the room and freeze when you turn around. If you spot anyone moving then they must go back to the beginning.

★ Anyone who reaches you without being seen can then become the BFG.

★ When in role as the BFG, use some of the unusual sounds and words from the story whenever you turn around to try and catch the group out, such as

'Winksquiffler' or 'Phizzwizard'. You could even add rules to the game so that when you say a different word they have to do something different, for example: when you say 'Winksquiffler' they have to freeze, when you say 'Trogglehumper' they have to sit down, and when you say 'Phizzwizard' they must all go back to the beginning.

Activity: Visiting Dream Country

★ Invite the group to join you on a journey to 'Dream Country', to find the cave where the BFG lives.

★ To get there the group must journey through different landscapes (such as grass, forest, mud or water, with actions to match). You can also ask the group to suggest the different modes of transport they might need to get there and then act out each suggestion e.g., taking a bus and then a boat over the sea. (You could use gym mats to create a contained space for the boat.)

★ Ask everyone if they can find a cave and once you have decided where it is, ask the group to form the shape of the cave with their bodies, all working together as a team. Allow each person in turn to leave the group shape and enter the cave.

Activity: Dream Jars

★ Gather the group in a circle and bring out the 'dream jars' you have prepared.

★ Tell the group that these jars contain dreams but you don't know what kind they are (it may be useful to read the section from the story before this exercise, where the BFG shows Sophie the dreams he collects in jars).

★ Ask the group to consider what kind of dream they think is inside each jar. Working in small groups, give everyone time to look, shake and explore the dream jars.

★ Ask each small group to decide what kind of dream they think is inside their jar and to develop actions and sounds that show what would happen if the jar was opened up and the dream let out.

For groups with lower support needs, encourage them to begin their 'Dream Piece' by making the shape of the jar with their bodies, with one or two people 'inside' as the dream. They then have to work out how their jar opens and what happens when the dream escapes. Finally, the dream has to return to the jar and the lid closes again to re-capture the dream. To encourage interaction between participants ask someone from another group to come and open up a dream jar when sharing the work in the larger group.

Activity: Dream Catching

★ Offer each participant a piece of coloured ribbon or length of tinsel, to represent a dream.

★ Put on some music that offers a sense of excitement and magic.

★ Encourage everyone to move their ribbon or tinsel to the music and dance in the space, as if they are 'catching dreams'.

★ Invite the group to work in pairs, attempting to catch each other's dreams by trying to gently catch the end of their partner's ribbon while it is moving.

★ Finally, come together again in the whole group in a circle and invite each 'dream' to dance in the centre of the circle. If everyone in the circle holds hands then the circle can represent a jar where the dream is held.

Activity: Making a Dream Potion

★ Once the dreams have all been caught, place a container such a bowl or bucket, into the centre of the circle (or an imaginary one if necessary) and invite each person to place their ribbon or 'dream' inside the container one at a time to make a 'dream potion'.

★ As each participant places their dream inside the container, give them a spoon (imaginary or real) to stir the mixture. As you do this, blow some bubbles over them as if their stirring is having an impact on the mixture.

Activity: Dream Sounds

★ Once all the dreams have been collected in the jar and the imaginary lid has been put on tightly, explain to the group that it is now time to find out what sounds each of their dreams make.

★ Using musical instruments and/or voices, ask each person to demonstrate what their dream sounds like. This should be a short and simple sound that can be repeated over and over again – something they can easily remember. For example (using instrument and voice): '*Shake, shake, whizzzzzzzzz! Shake, shake, whizzzzzzzzzzzzz!*'

★ Once everyone in the circle has created their sound, tell the group that it is time to hear the sounds of the dream potion they have created.

★ Pretend to slowly unscrew the lid of the container holding the 'Dream Potion'. As you take the lid off, everyone should create their chosen sound, repeating it over and over again.

★ You can halt the sound at any time by replacing the lid on the jar. Remind the group to watch you carefully in order for this to be successful (this can become a group game of watching and listening.)

If working with people with visual impairments, you can create a sound cue to indicate when you have replaced the lid of the jar, such as a clap.

Activity: Return Journey

★ Once the group has completed making their dream potion, tell them that it is time to leave Dream Country. (You could even suggest that they leave their potion as a gift for the BFG when he returns to his cave).

★ Leave the 'cave' and get the group to retrace their steps, remembering (in reverse order) how they got there.

★ Gather the group back into a circle and get them to speak, gesture or sign their favourite part of the experience of visiting Dream Country.

FURTHER DEVELOPMENT

Undoubtedly the theme of dreams is one that would be meaningful to groups of any age. However, whether working with adults or children it is important to note the potentially sensitive nature of this subject, as dreams are incredibly personal and often deeply meaningful. It is therefore worth saying to the group that they should only share what they feel comfortable with and create a clear plan and structure for such work. The aim of this theme is not to create a therapeutic session exploring people's unconscious processes, but to give participants a space in which to consider what dreams mean to them. You can explore the theme of dreams without even touching on people's personal dream scenarios.

The following activity could be used to explore the theme of dreams with any group of children or adults. Also bear in mind that a number of the activities already discussed could be adapted for use with adult groups, regardless of whether the group are familiar with the actual BFG story.

Activity: The Dream Tree

★ On a large piece of paper draw the outline of a big tree with long branches that can be stuck up on a wall and tell the group it is to become a 'Dream Tree'.

★ Give everyone in the group some sticky notes (or pre-cut paper leaves) and ask them to write or draw responses to the statement 'A dream is…'

★ Each new idea should be put on a separate sticky note or leaf and stuck up on the branches of the tree.

★ Once all of the leaves have been stuck on the tree, gather everyone around and read out all of the responses.

★ Now invite people to select a few of the responses from the tree (either their own or someone else's) to work with in small groups. To make this process fair you could invite participants to come up in any order and select one note that appeals to them. If you have two people wanting the same words or statement then write it out again on a separate note.

CASE STUDY

EXAMPLES OF RESPONSES FROM DREAM CATCHERS PROJECT

A Dream is…

Enormous or small

A game

Skipping through flowers

Unicorns, dragons, skeletons

Invisible

Hopeful

Magic and spine-tingling

Big, bigger and bigger!

Flying and jumping

My sister being nice to me

Terribly scary and frightening

Extreme

Something you can't see unless you know it in your head

★ The groups now need to create a short movement piece that incorporates all of their chosen words and statements. Encourage them to use sound and words if they wish. If you have time, the whole group could create a soundscape using instruments and voice that could even be recorded and played back to help support each piece.

★ Get each small group to share their work with the whole group in turn.

If working with people with limited mobility, you could use pieces of material or ribbons that they can move easily. Words and statements from the Dream Tree could also be explored using tableaux and sound rather than movement. If you have the materials and time at the end of the session, you could invite everyone to draw or paint an image that captures the essence of their piece.

Working with Teenage Groups
Romeo & Juliet

ORIGINAL SETTING

This workshop was developed as part of a programme introducing teenagers with special needs to Shakespeare and was designed to have flexibility both with regards to the needs of the group and the spaces in which the workshop would take place (from large sports halls to intimate classrooms).

Over the years it has been used with a variety of ages and disabilities including young people with emotional and behavioural difficulties, those with autism spectrum disorders, mobility impairments and complex disabilities. It is also an ideal workshop for groups that include a wide mix of needs including non-disabled participants.

It was originally planned as a one-off workshop lasting approximately ninety minutes, however, it has since provided the basis for developing theatre productions of 'Romeo & Juliet' and as a springboard into term-long projects on subjects such as love, friendship, parent-child relationships and gang culture.

THE WORKSHOP

Props & Materials

You will need:

★ A whistle

★ A collection of half-face masks in two colours

★ A selection of music both for dancing and 'mirroring'

Activity: Insults

★ Introduce the concept of two families at war. Explain that this has been going on for generations, has divided the community and harsh penalties are in place for anyone caught fighting.

★ Split the group into two sides (the Montagues and Capulets) and have them line up facing each other, a distance apart, on opposite sides of the room.

★ Using call and response, ask the groups to use the following dialogue (adapted from the original text) to create a chant. Action and stamping can go with the rhythm, but stress that both groups must stay on the spot until directed to do otherwise.

For those with limited speech or mobility, drums and other percussion instruments can be included as an accompaniment to the spoken word.

MONTAGUE:	Do you bite your thumb at us?
CAPULET:	Bite my thumb?
MONTAGUE:	Do you bite your thumb at us?
CAPULET:	Bite my thumb?
MONTAGUE:	Quarrel, sir?
CAPULET:	No, sir.
MONTAGUE:	You do, sir.
CAPULET:	No.
MONTAGUE:	Lie.
CAPULET:	Draw!

Ultimately the call-and-response rhythm should go something like this:

> Do you bite your thumb at us? (Do you bite your thumb at us?)
>
> Bite my thumb? (Bite my thumb?)
>
> Do you bite your thumb at us? (Do you bite your thumb at us?)
>
> Bite my thumb? (Bite my thumb?)
>
> Quarrel, sir? (Quarrel, sir?)
>
> No, sir! (No, sir!)
>
> You do, sir! (You do, sir!)
>
> No! (No!)
>
> Lie. (Lie.)
>
> Draw!

★ On 'Draw!' have both groups freeze in position and get them all to take one step towards each other.

★ Repeat the call and response rhythm, building intensity, increasing the pace and volume until they reach 'Draw!' again. Have the groups take another step towards each other and repeat the process yet again. Eventually they should be standing about an arms length apart.

★ As the group says their final 'Draw!' blow the whistle and in role as Escalus (the Prince and law-maker of Verona) send both groups back to their original position.

★ Maintaining your role, reiterate that fighting is outlawed and that you have the ultimate power to stop the celebration party that the Capulets are holding that night.

While in-role, sow the seeds of the story by insisting that the Montagues stay away from the party and any other information you feel is needed.
For example:

> *"I don't want to see any of you Montagues at the Capulet's party tonight.*
> *Romeo, Mercutio – stay out of trouble. Capulets, I don't want any trouble*

from you either. Tybalt, remember it's Juliet's party – not yours. For too long your families have been at war, so from now on the penalty is death to anyone caught disturbing the peace."

★ Drop role as Escalus and prompt a discussion on what just happened. Questions could include:

    – Was the penalty handed down by Escalus fair?

    – What would they do to maintain the peace?

    – Whose fault is it that the families are fighting?

Note: If you have a group prone to actual fighting, instead of moving towards each other, this activity could be staged with both groups seated and standing up on 'Draw!' either as a group or one at a time.

Activity: *The Masked Ball*

★ While you work with the Montagues, have a support worker plan the party with the Capulets, deciding on favourite foods, what they might wear or do at the party and distributing masks (of all one colour) for them to wear.

If no support worker is available, let both groups (out of role) be involved in both the planning of the party and coming up with ideas of how to 'gatecrash' it. Although not ideal, it can be beneficial to have both groups work together for this initial activity.

★ Working with the Montagues, ask them if they think they should try and go to the party, and to suggest ideas for how to get in unseen.

CASE STUDY

At no time in any of the workshops did I have a group of Montagues not wanting to go to the party and when prompted for ways of getting in, they always came up with the idea of wearing masks. Although I was leading them towards this idea anyway, it was important for them to discover it for themselves, as it not only helped to build belief in the imagined world, but allowed them to start claiming ownership of the work.

★ Give out the masks of the other colour to the Montagues, reiterating that 'We're going to go to their ball wearing masks so they don't recognise us.'

★ Play some dance music to start the party and instruct the group that when the music stops they must freeze.

★ On the first 'freeze' take on the role of Lord Capulet saying in a loud voice,

"I have been told that there may be Montagues at this party. So we will test the guests to see if this is true".

Should any Capulets deliberately point out a Montague, state that your old traditional test will catch them out and that you will need their help to make sure it is done properly.

★ Tell the group to each find a partner with a different coloured mask from their own, help them to pair up if necessary, i.e., a Capulet opposite a Montague.

★ Change the music to something slower. Tell the Capulets to move to the music while the person opposite them has to copy their movements as closely as possible (remind the Montagues that they don't want to be caught).

★ After a short time, fade the music and in-role thank the Capulets, saying that so far you haven't seen any Montagues but will keep an eye out for them.

★ Return to the dance music and encourage the group to dance.

★ Repeat the mirroring 'test' exercise a few more times before discovering that indeed there are Montagues at the party.

★ Explain that you want no trouble and have both groups return to their respective sides.

Activity: The Balcony Scene

★ Out of role, ask Romeo (on the Montague side) to stand up. If no Romeo has been established by now, ask who would like to play the part.

★ Ask Juliet (on the Capulet side) to also stand up.

CASE STUDY

Often the roles of Romeo, Juliet and the supporting cast would have been established during the preliminary Masked Ball activities. Again, this was never something I initiated, but would often happen spontaneously. The only obstacle I once had was when working in an all-boys school as they didn't want to cast anyone as Juliet. So during the Balcony Scene, I took on the role myself, stepping in to mirror Romeo while a support worker conducted the group.

★ Bring Romeo and Juliet into the centre of the room and ask them to repeat the mirroring exercise. This could potentially be embarrassing so before asking them to move, introduce the activity. For example, 'During the Capulet party, Romeo and Juliet met for the first time and started dancing'.

★ Put the slow music back on and ask them to repeat the mirroring exercise (you may find that if they continue to wear the masks this will help to counteract any embarrassment).

★ While they're moving, go up to the Montagues and ask for Romeo's friend Mercutio. Ask Mercutio what he thinks of Romeo dancing with Juliet. Does he think it's a good thing or a bad thing? What would he like to say to his friend?

★ Invite Mercutio to stand up and speak aloud his thoughts to Romeo, over and over (this could be a continuous stream of thoughts, one word, a sound or even a repeatable action). There is no right or wrong for this discourse and it doesn't even have to coincide with the original play, as who is to say that Mercutio didn't encourage Romeo in this affair or even find himself jealous?

★ Pause the action and ask for Lord Capulet from the other group. Ask him what he thinks of his daughter dancing with a Montague.

★ Start Romeo and Juliet's mirroring exercise again, bringing in Mercutio's repeatable opinions followed by Lord Capulet repeating his views. The effect should be that of a sound orchestra with you as the conductor.

★ Bring to a stop and repeat the process with other characters from each group (such as the Nurse, Tybalt, Benvolio, Friar Lawrence and so forth) until everyone is involved in a cacophony of orchestrated sound.

★ Once completed, ask Romeo and Juliet how they felt having these many and varied opinions shouted out at them.

Activity: *Completing The Story*

★ Keeping everyone in their positions from the previous activity, bring characters forward to create frozen (tableau) images of the following as you narrate the remainder of the story. For example:

★ 'Ignoring everyone's advice, Romeo and Juliet escaped their parents and went to Friar Lawrence to get married.'

★ 'While this was going on, Tybalt and Mercutio fought a duel. Romeo arrived just in time to see Tybalt kill Mercutio.' (A slow-motion fight could occur that ends with another frozen image.)

★ 'Romeo was so enraged that he killed Tybalt.'

★ 'Romeo was banished from Verona forever.'

★ 'Juliet was so distressed that she took poison to kill herself.'

★ 'Romeo heard of Juliet's death and was so distraught that he took his own life.'

CASE STUDY

Although we deliberately simplified the ending, sometimes groups knew the story and would correct us, staging the moment Juliet would awaken only to discover her Romeo dead beside her.

When we first did this workshop, our final image was that of four dead bodies (Romeo, Juliet, Mercutio and Tybalt). I then turned to both Lord Capulet and Lord Montague and told them to look closely at the carnage their war had created, asking 'What do you think should happen now?' Without any warning the two boys walked towards each other and shook hands. Thinking it was a fluke, I didn't want to deliberately prompt it for future workshops, however, the shaking of hands continued in subsequent sessions, becoming a beautiful image with which to end the workshop.

FURTHER DEVELOPMENT

Following on from 'The Balcony Scene' activity, comments from those playing Romeo and Juliet often included feelings of being confused, upset and wanting to run away. These comments can provide a wonderful starting point for work on isolation, gangs and bullying behaviour, using drama techniques such as forum theatre to explore these issues further.

Groups might also like to make their own masks in preparation for the party and even spend time cooking food and playing other games.

'The Balcony Scene' activity is also a good structure for exploring any story, new or established. For example, giving advice to both Grandma and the Wolf in 'Little Red Riding Hood' and Kate and Petruchio in 'Taming of the Shrew'.

Working with Adults with Learning Disabilities

The Falling Star

ORIGINAL SETTING

Inspired by the Ted Hughes short story 'The Dancers', the following workshop was originally designed to help develop a theatre production with an adult drama group who met for two hours once a week. The ages in the group ranged from 17 to over 50 years and the needs were a mixture of autism, Downs Syndrome and general speech and language difficulties.

Prior to this show, the group had mainly worked on re-staging popular musicals and so the emphasis for this production was on devising an original story for an ensemble cast. Each activity was used to not only develop the story but as a theatrical device that could be repeated on-stage. In this way, members of the group who were often sidelined were able to fully participate in the show. Certain activities were also adapted to include audience participation.

Each of the activities was explored in a single two hour session.

THE WORKSHOP

Props & Materials

You will need:

★ A large piece of brown lycra material

★ A yellow or orange beach-ball

★ A selection of music (suggestion: Ladysmith Black Mambazo)

★ Torches (optional)

★ Two chairs

★ Rain-sticks and other shakers

★ A sword

★ A toy fish

★ A star that can be split in two

★ A large piece of blue material

★ Bubble pots (or a bubble-blowing machine)

★ Crown for the King of the Forest (optional)

★ A cape or hat to denote the role of the Wizard

★ A large cardboard box (painted black)

Activity: The Falling Star

★ Spread out the large piece of brown lycra material on the floor and ask the group to sit around the edges.

★ Play some music to help set the scene.

★ Dim the lights (if possible) and read the following excerpt from 'The Dancers'.

A great, flaming star was falling.

Owl looked up and the ball of fire, with its long tail, was reflected in their bulging eyes.

Most falling stars burn out to nothing, before they get near the earth. But this one did not. And the wide eyes of the Owls widened wider as the flaming ball grew and grew and – plunged silently into the dark mountains.

★ Create a soundscape with individuals repeating certain words or phrases from the above excerpt (or sounds inspired by it).

★ If possible, give out torches, darken the room and invite the group to repeat their chosen words or phrases (underscored with music) while torchlight is flashed around the room.

★ Finally, bring the lights back up and place the beach-ball in the centre of the brown material. Ask the group to hold the edges of the material and gently move the ball around the edges of material. As they become more confident working as a group in this way, the ball could start to bounce into the air and be caught again by the material.

If possible, try layering the above activities, so that while some of the group uses the torches, the others manipulate the beach-ball around the material. If speaking lines while doing this is too much then you could record people's voices to play back over the music.

★ To finish, wrap the beach-ball up in the brown material as you repeat the opening excerpt from the story.

Activity: News Arrives

★ Ask the group to create a busy village community with activities such as those mentioned in 'The Last Drummer' workshop.

★ Once established, introduce the dilemma of the Falling Star.

★ In role, discuss with the group what should be done (see 'The Sleeping Boy' workshop for more ideas on how to develop a quest). Questions to help prompt could include:

– Why do you think the star has fallen?

– Should we go and look for it?

– How will the star falling out of the sky affect our village?

CASE STUDY

Although the person introducing the dilemma in our group could speak, he came up with a way of giving news of the falling star non-verbally. As he entered the village, the music they were working to faded. He then raised his hand high into the air and brought it down slowly. He did this three times before the rest of the group copied his movement.

The group also decided that an evil wizard had cast a spell, causing the star to not only fall but split into two separate pieces. Therefore two people from the village would go in opposite directions to find the separate fragments.

Activity: Leaving Gifts

★ Ask everyone to think of a parting gift or piece of advice they would give to those going on the quest.

★ Place two chairs at the far end of the room and create a tunnel for the two journeying villagers to walk through (this could be done with group members' bodies or with material and pieces of furniture). Play some music to help add to the sense of ritual and occasion.

★ Once they have walked through the tunnel, they can sit on the chairs while each member of the village comes forward and presents them with their parting gift and/or piece of advice.

Once everyone has presented their gift, they should sit facing the chairs. Ask the two people questions on their impending journey. (These questions can also be adapted and asked of the villagers watching.) For example:

– How do you feel knowing that you will be leaving your village?

– Are you worried about the journey ahead?

– Is there anything you would like to say to the villagers before you go?

For those with autism spectrum disorders, the separation between themselves and their character might need more definition, so the question could be re-phrased in the third person, for example "How do you think your character might be feeling now?" Alternatively, you might like to give definite choices such as, "Do you think your character is feeling brave or scared?"

If you have some members in the group who are non-verbal, use a 'Master of Ceremonies' to announce the arrival of each member of the village and state their gift. Not only does this include everyone in the drama but it also helps to create a sense of occasion.

Activity: The Forest of Darkness

★ Narrate the following: "As s/he travelled, s/he came to the edge of a forest."

★ Give the group a selection of rain-sticks and other shakers. Slowly conduct them into creating a soundscape of the forest.

★ Ask one of the people on the quest to start to walk through the forest (created by the rest of the group).

★ As they walk through, the soundscape starts and the trees they have passed slowly follow them. However, should the person on the quest turn around, the sound should suddenly stop and the forest freeze.

★ Eventually the King of the Forest appears and the following dialogue ensues:

King:	STOP!
Villager:	I'm looking for a star.
King:	What's the password?
Villager:	I don't know.

King: You have five guesses.

Villager: Is the password [_____]?

King: NO!

Villager: Is the password [_____]?

King: NO!

Villager: Is the password [_____]?

King: NO! You have two guesses left.

Suddenly the good spirit of the forest enters and hands the villager a sword and a fish.

Villager: Is the password 'fishsword'?

King: NO!

The spirit signals for him to switch the words around.

Villager: Is the password 'swordfish'?

King: YES!

★ As the King of the Forest presents the villager with half of the fallen star the forest can recap their soundscape.

CASE STUDY

In the show, the actor playing the villager allowed for some audience participation, by turning to the audience and asking for people's names, trying them out as the first three guesses of the password.

It could transpire that the villager becomes entombed within the trees and needs to be rescued by someone. Or maybe he defends himself with an axe or performs a heroic deed that earns him the respect of the forest inhabitants.

Activity: The Lake

★ Narrate the following: "As s/he travelled s/he came to the edge of a lake."

★ Spread out the large blue material, with two people holding either end. Play some music as the material is wafted high into the air for the group to 'swim' beneath.

★ Once everyone has been swimming, the Queen of the Mermaids appears and the following dialogue ensues.

Queen:	You can't pass.
Villager:	I'm looking for the star.
Queen:	You must pass the test.
Villager:	What is it?
Queen:	Copy me.

★ Play some music while the questing villager copies the movements of the Queen and the remainder of the group blow bubbles.

★ Once completed, fade the music as the Queen of the Mermaids presents the villager with the other half of the fallen star and the group repeats the activity of running under the blue material.

Activity: The Wizard's Plan

★ Narrate the following: "Deep inside the mountain the wizard was hard at work."

★ Spend some time developing the wizard's lair. This can be done in a number of ways, including:

– Creating an actual den.

– Drawing pictures of what the den might look like.

– Asking individuals to mime actions of what might be in the room or what the wizard might get up to. For example, stirring a cauldron, reading a book, feeding the rats or casting a spell.

★ Cast someone to play the wizard. Place them in a chair in front of the group and 'hotseat' them, asking questions such as:

– Why would you steal the star?

– Did you know it would break into pieces?

– What do you think of the villagers who have gone looking for the star?

While this scene is being improvised, the rest of the group can become the wizard's guard, learning how to march and stand at attention. The wizard can then call individuals forward and give them commands. This could become an adaptation of the 'Simon Says' game. Eventually the wizard should give the order to cast a spell.

★ Once the wizard's plan has been discovered, cast a spell with the group (this can be done with movement, music, chants or a combination of techniques to create a ritual).

★ While the spell is taking place, narrate the following, guiding the two villagers in the process.

"Gradually the spell began to work. As if pulled by an invisible thread, the two villagers and their star fragments began to walk, very slowly, towards the mountain. Towards the wizard's lair."

CASE STUDY

The spell could have different effects depending on the choices made. For example, it might have been designed to shatter the star fragments (in which case they might have then been light enough to fly back up into the sky). Or the group might decide to keep the world in darkness, so the village must find their own source of light (generating electricity or discovering fire for the first time).

★ Once they are in position, create a final tableau with the villagers, guards and wizard.

★ Discuss with the group what they think might happen next.

Activity: The Star Fragments

★ Bring out the large black box, with the orange beach-ball hidden inside.

★ Ceremoniously hand the box to the person playing the wizard, guiding the action with dialogue such as, "Here sir, is the box you ordered. It should be able to contain the star fragments so they can't escape."

★ With the group all sitting in a circle, play some music (or the group could start a slow drum beat) as the two star fragments are slowly brought together. If possible, ask the two villagers what they might say or do in that situation and let them shout their protests over the music and/or rhythm as the star fragments are being brought together.

★ Once the two star fragments are in the box, stop all sound and in the silence, place the box in the centre of the room, narrating the following.

"The world was dark. The mountains were silent. Nobody moved. It appeared that the wizard had won ... when suddenly there was a sound. The big black box was moving, was shaking, was stirring. The wizard looked as the box opened. The wizard looked as the two star fragments became whole once more, shining light high into the air. Lighting up the mountains and the sky. The wizard retreated. He had failed. Cursing he went back into his lair deep inside the mountain. He would return, but for now the people were happy. They rejoiced, and the star ... danced."

★ Slowly lift the orange beach-ball out of the box, raise it high into the air and bounce it around the group.

FURTHER DEVELOPMENT

★ Time could be spent making or drawing the parting gifts given to the journeying villagers.

★ On their return, the villagers could re-tell the story of their journey, and this could be drawn as a timeline of events or recreated in dance or song.

★ As the original story involves animals, the group could play at being different animals. Explorations could include movement, sound and how each animal is affected by day and night.

Working in Adult Care Settings
The Return of the Flowers

ORIGINAL SETTING

This workshop was a one-off storytelling session at a hospice for people with terminal illness and was to take place as part of an activities week. The hospice had never had a storytelling workshop before and so preparation was needed to ensure that all the necessary requirements were put in place, such as a safe space, good support and access to the necessary equipment. The workshop was to run for two- and a-half-hours with up to twelve participants. All the participants had a terminal illness and their ages ranged from 45 to 70 years old. This workshop is therefore written with this particular group in mind, however, all the activities described can be adapted for use with a group of older adults or people of any age or needs.

PREPARATION

It was not known whether the participants had previous experience of drama work or how many would be interested in attending on the day, but the hope was that the workshop would not only engage participants in creative activity but also offer some therapeutic value. Using a multisensory approach as a starting point, the workshop intended to offer participants the opportunity to go on an imaginative journey into the world of a traditional story, as well as have the chance to share and tell their own stories if they wished.

The story of 'The Return of the Flowers' is an ancient Australian Aboriginal myth which was chosen carefully for its symbols and themes in relation to the setting in which the workshop was taking place. When working in a hospice or care home for older adults, try to choose a story that will resonate with the participants without being too direct or heavy. This particular story seemed to offer a sense of hope through its focus on colour, new life and nature, while still symbolically exploring the themes of change and loss. There can be a tendency, especially when working with older adults, to focus predominantly on the past through reminiscence. When working with people coming towards the end of their lives, it is important to offer an opportunity to reflect on the present and future, as well as the past.

In the workshop plan that follows, you will see that your role as storyteller becomes more fixed, as you are telling (and re-telling) a narrative which you need to know well. One of the most successful aspects of this workshop was that it offered the group a new creative experience. The use of tactile and sensory objects (in particular the flowers, plants and stones) seemed to have a strong impact on the group. Many commented on how the experience allowed them to really appreciate what was around them (one woman reflected that the activity had inspired her to go back to her own garden and look more closely at what was growing there). Very often, creative activity in care settings helps people to find ways of communicating and socialising with those around them. Hospices and care homes can be isolating places at times and so this kind of work can make a real difference.

Working with any vulnerable group raises certain challenges that need thought before you begin this kind of activity. The one-off nature of such a workshop may mean that there is some anxiety about what the group are expected to do. People may be concerned that they will be expected to 'act', especially those unfamiliar with story or drama work. Reassure the group from the outset that their level of involvement is completely at their discretion and that there is no right or wrong way to do it.

If you have time to develop a sense of playfulness and spontaneity with the group beforehand, then you should find that their participation comes much more easily when you initiate it. Try to create and choose activities according to how familiar the group are with drama and also how well they know each other; if the group are completely new to drama work and do not know each other at all, then keep things very simple and comfortable. You don't want to throw them in at the deep end and scare them off. However, there can also be some benefit in encouraging people to take risks and work outside their comfort zone, if you feel it is right for them.

You should find that the group's uncertainty will disperse once the story is under way and there will also be a natural tendency for people to join in even if they had previously shown resistance. It is vital to acknowledge any small contribution to the storytelling and you may well find that someone who only appears willing to shake an instrument in the first few moments of the story, takes on a significant role at a later stage. Very often at the end of a workshop experience, there will be a great sense of celebration arising from the fact that the group have taken a risk and participated in something they have never done before. As long as your group feels safe in the knowledge that no-one will laugh at or judge them, then taking risks can be both exciting and satisfying.

What follows is a workshop structure that contains activities which link directly to the themes of the chosen story. By looking at the themes and symbols within a story, you can develop a variety of creative ideas that help the participants connect with it on a deeper level when it is told. Furthermore, the story may develop and change as the group begins to work with it. Don't be afraid to go with the group's ideas, even if this means the story changing entirely; there will be a reason for doing this that is meaningful to the group, so it is important to go with it. What can become difficult is when some participants alter the direction of the story while others seem put out by this. In such a situation it is possible to enact two versions of the story, one after the other, and discuss the impact these different versions have on the group. It is always useful to leave time at the end to reflect on what has happened and to allow individuals to share their thoughts and feelings about the session as a whole.

The Return Of The Flowers – Story

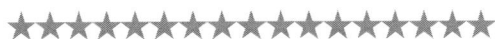

★★★★★★★★★★★★★★★★★★★★

Baiame, the Great One, remained for a long while on earth as a man and made his home in the mountains. Around the mountains and across the earth, flowers bloomed in brilliant colours and trees blossomed, constantly bursting with fruit. The whole earth was full of brilliant colour and light because of Baiame's presence, which made the people feel peaceful and happy.

One day Baiame called the humans and animals to him and said: 'The time has come for me to leave you… while the earth was young, you needed me but now you are fully grown, it is better you are by yourself.' There was a low moan of disappointment, but Baiame smiled and told them not to be sad. He explained that the time had now come when he must return to his home in the sky. Before Baiame departed, he informed the animals and humans that if they ever needed him he would be there. And with that Baiame was gone.

The animals and people lay down on the multi-coloured carpet and breathed in the smell of the sweet perfume, whilst looking up at the Sky to where the Great One now lived. Soon the people became uncomfortable and they did not know why. They looked about them and suddenly one woman cried out: 'The flowers have gone!' As they looked, they saw that the bright green leaves and white blossom were falling from the trees, the bees were falling to the ground and the flowers were drooping. Soon there were no flowers left anywhere. The earth became bare and brown because Baiame had gone to his home in the Sky.

Much time passed and the earth remained colourless and bare. The people who were able to remember the flowers and trees grieved for what had been lost and told stories to their children about how it had been.

One day, a group of wise Elders decided to journey to Baiame to plead with him to return the trees and flowers to the earth. They set off towards the foot of the mountains and found a path of stone steps leading up the mountain. They climbed for four days and four nights, unwilling to rest until they reached the summit. At the top they lay down exhausted, unsure where to go next or what to do. All of a sudden, one of the Elders noticed in the distance stones formed in the shape of a circle. Feeling their spirits rising again they made their way towards the stone circle. As they stood within the stones, they heard the voice of Baiame calling to them, and then felt themselves being lifted up into the Sky.

As they looked about them, tears streamed down their faces as they saw what lay before them – a carpet of the most beautiful colours and flowers, more vibrant than they had ever seen. Wherever Baiame was, flowers and trees bloomed eternally. Baiame saw the tears on the faces of his people and realised why they had come to him. He knew they had fought a long and arduous journey to return flowers to the earth.

So Baiame told the people to gather armfuls of flowers and tree shoots, as many as they could carry, and scatter them across the earth. Once their arms were full to bursting, Baiame's gentle hand carried the Elders back through the Stone Circle and onto the mountain top where they had come from.

The Elders journeyed back down the mountain and ran to their tribes, dropping flowers as they went and scattering the colours all around. The people on earth who had never before seen flowers or trees gazed in awe at the beautiful colours and smelled the sweet fragrances. Once more, trees and flowers graced the earth, filling the hearts of the people with hope and joy.

(Abridged by Rosie Emanuel from two versions of the story: Reed, 1994, *Aboriginal Stories* and Gersie, 1990, *Storymaking in Education and Therapy*.)

STORY STRUCTURE

Props & Materials

You will need:

★ A table with a cloth

★ A range of flower and plant stems with a variety of shape, texture, colour and scent (if you have access to a garden you should find a huge variety when you look closely)

★ A range of colourful ribbons, each about half a metre in length

★ A large piece of lycra (preferably green)

★ A multi-coloured soft sensory ball (or equivalent)

★ A range of musical instruments – enough for each person

★ Some gentle instrumental music

★ A CD player

★ A range of art and craft materials

Set up the room so that all of the flower and plant stems are laid out on the table ready to be explored. It is useful to have the musical instruments in a basket which can be taken round for people to choose from. Make sure that the CD player is easily accessible for you to turn on and off where necessary.

Activity: Welcome/Sign Names

★ Once the group is seated in a circle, welcome them into the space and explain a little about what the session will involve. At this point it is a good idea to explain that the group can participate as much or as little as they wish and that there is no right or wrong way of doing things. Now play a game which will help to put the group at ease.

★ One opening activity which works well, especially if the group don't know each other, is to invite each person to say their name and then create an action or 'sign name' which represents something about their character. For example, if someone enjoys playing the violin, they may say their name and then mime this action (adding sound if possible). Alternatively it could be an action to represent an aspect of their character, such as 'friendly' or 'disorganised'.

★ Now the whole group should echo the action back together and then move on to the next person. Once everyone has created their action, challenge the group to remember each one by doing them all again quickly in sequence. The sign-names could then be used as an opening ritual every week if working regularly with a group.

★ A variation on creating sign-names is to invite each person to say their name plus anything that they know about the history of their name, or why it was chosen for them. This allows people to share a little personal information about themselves, without it feeling too invasive.

Activity: Lycra Platform

★ Bring a piece of lycra to the circle and ask the group to stretch it from one side to another. Make sure that everyone is making contact with the material with both hands if possible. It should look like a 'platform' at about chest level; you can play around with the levels, getting the group to try lifting it above their heads to create a 'sky' and then down low, without letting it go.

★ Once the lycra is secure in its place across the circle, place the ball on top and let it roll around. The group must work as a team to try and keep the ball on top of the lycra. If it falls off the edge it really doesn't matter – just pick it up and put it back on. Once the group have got the hang of this, try throwing the ball up into the air, using the lycra like a trampoline, but make sure the ball is soft enough to not be a hazard when it comes back down!

Activity: Ribbons

★ Once the group feel a little more at ease with each other, introduce the ribbons. This activity is best done in a seated circle so that everyone can see each other clearly, although feel free to try moving around the space. Invite each person to choose a ribbon by offering a selection and then to explore its shape, flexibility and movements. Now invite each participant to share a movement they have discovered with their ribbon, which everyone else can copy.

★ Play some appropriate music that might inspire movement and invite the group to explore the shapes and patterns their piece of ribbon makes. Then get them to interact with others in the group, creating 'ribbon dances' in pairs.

★ If moving about the space, ask them to try and 'meet' every other ribbon in the room. You may also like to encourage a variety of speed in their movements, as well as exploring different levels. The variety of colour and movement from the ribbons should create a beautiful image. Later in the session, the group will come to realise that their ribbons represent the colours of the flowers in the story.

CASE STUDY

Using ribbons as a tool is a fantastic way of developing movement and dance skills, as the ribbons inspire new and different styles of movement in the body. You can get the participants to work in small groups and to choreograph their own 'ribbon dance' where they must use a variety of movement styles: fast and slow, high and low, big and small, etc. They can then perform their pieces to music in front of their peers.

Activity: Sand Leader

★ Once the group have had a chance to explore the use of ribbons in this way, stop the music and invite them all to choose a percussion instrument from the basket. Now, working with a partner (who may be the person next to them), ask them to choose one person to use their ribbon and one to use their instrument.

★ The person using the instrument is the leader and as they explore the sounds of their instrument, the person with the ribbon must respond to the sounds being made and alter their movements accordingly. Once one person has had a go at leading with their sounds, let them swap over so that the other person has a chance to lead.

Using musical instruments at this point in the session will help the group become familiar with them, as they might be needed later during the storytelling. It is also a useful exercise in communication and interaction.

Activity: Sensory Exploration of Flowers

★ Collect the ribbons and instruments and place the table containing the flower and plant stems in the centre of the circle. You could also start your background music at this point.

★ Ask everyone to come up to the table and choose a stem. Invite them to share with their neighbour what they find interesting or unusual about the plant or whether they know what kind it might be.

★ Once they have shared their first choice of stem, ask everyone to pass their chosen plant to the person next to them, until everyone has had a chance to explore each one.

★ Encourage the group to touch and smell the plants and to share with others anything of particular interest. Perhaps the plants evoke a memory or story which can be shared? Leave space and opportunity for this to happen if you feel there are some interesting ideas coming out of the sensory experience.

★ If you are working with a group over a number of weeks, you could use this sensory flower exercise to create a whole session, without needing to move straight into the storytelling. The flowers and plants may inspire the group to share memories or stories of their own, which could then be used to create a piece of movement, music, drama or artwork. You could even have a go at inviting the group to write a poem inspired by the plants. The rest of the workshop could then be spread over the next few sessions.

Activity: Telling the Story

★ Ask everyone to place the flowers and plants back in the centre of the table and tell them that you are now going to tell them the story of 'The Return of the Flowers'.

Some notes on telling the story:

★ Engage with the group using good eye contact;

★ Try to keep the storytelling to no more than 10 minutes in length;

★ Speak clearly and try not to rush, making sure that anyone with a hearing impairment sits close to you;

★ Make a point of starting and ending the story with a few moments of quiet;

★ At the end you might want to close with a phrase such as: '… and that is the story of The Return of the Flowers', so that everyone knows it has finished.

★ Once the storytelling has ended, invite the group to think about which particular parts of the story interested them and which characters they were drawn to. Allow them to discuss this either with the whole group or a partner.

Activity: The Retelling

★ Explain that with the group's help you will be acting out the story and remind them that their involvement can be as simple as making small sounds. Ensure that the group knows that they can do whatever they feel comfortable with, and that they can join in and play a part at anytime, even if it is not something they originally chose. (Welcome them warmly if someone suddenly feels inclined to become part of the mountain, for example!)

★ Now ask each individual to share which character from the story they are drawn to; this might be a human or animal character or perhaps an object such as the flowers or mountain. It is important to note that two people might want to play one part together, which is fine. In fact, this can be actively encouraged, as it can be reassuring to know you won't be alone in a part, especially if drama and storytelling is new to you.

★ Invite the group to use any of the objects or props to help them (they will now be familiar with the ribbons, flowers and instruments) which are likely to be useful and effective tools in the retelling of the story.

> ## CASE STUDY
>
> In one workshop, most of the participants spontaneously used their ribbons to represent the return of the flowers at the end, creating a dazzling array of coloured movement in the circle.

From here, the enactment should be spontaneous and playful. You will narrate the story again from the beginning and will facilitate as characters come into the centre of the circle (or enact a part from their chair if preferable). You might have to narrate and act a part at the same time, or you can request that a support worker takes on numerous roles.

It is important to ensure that *someone* takes on the main role of Baiame (suggested pronunciation: *Bay-a-me*), even if it is you or a support worker. This character can be represented by a cloak worn around the shoulders, which could be passed around so that different people have a chance to play the part if they wish.

★ As the story enactment progresses, adapt your narration according to what you see. It may be that the people playing the Elders show great exhaustion climbing the mountain, so narrate this. The group may not realise it, but you will often be responding to *them*, rather than them having to follow you and 'act out' what you are saying. However, as the narrator it is your job to keep the story *moving*.

This type of enactment can be challenging for a new group and is something that you may need to work up to over a number of weeks. The best advice is to maintain a sense of playfulness, while showing respect to the story and its meaning.

Participants may simply mime their involvement, leaving yours as the only spoken voice in the room.

Activity: Reflection

★ Once the retelling of the story is complete, give everyone a chance come back into the circle and share any thoughts or feelings about their experience.

★ Put on some music and lay out some art materials on a table; try to include a variety of different materials such as paints, craft objects, pencils and charcoals.

This activity gives everyone time to reflect on their own, or socially with others, through the creation of images inspired by the story. Invite the group to draw, paint or make anything that they like; it could be a memory of a moment in the story or an image of something they want to remember.

Activity: Ending

★ Gather back in a circle and give the group a chance to share their images (if they want to) and to add any final thoughts or comments about the story or the session.

★ If you are working over a number of weeks, use a ritual to close the session such as a song or a simple game; you could even repeat the opening 'sign-name' exercise, going around the circle one final time to say goodbye to each person individually.

FURTHER DEVELOPMENT

★ Try exploring the environment of the story. Get the group to decide where in the room each part of the story takes place. One corner might be the village where the people live, another might be the mountains and another the sky. Explore the different environments through soundscape and/or artwork.

★ Take some key moments from the story and divide into small groups, inviting each group to recreate one moment using movement or still images. To aid this, prepare some pieces of paper describing the key moments of the story. Give one to each group and then, as you narrate the story, ask each group to share their images or movement piece at the relevant time.

Further Reading

Campbell, J., 1991, *The Power of Myth*, Anchor Books

Cattanach, A., 1997, *Children's Stories in Play Therapy*, Jessica Kingsley Publishers

Crimmens, P., 2006, *Drama Therapy and Storymaking in Special Education*, Jessica Kingsley Publishers

Crimmens, P., 1998, *Storymaking and Creative Groupwork with Older People*, Jessica Kingsley Publishers

Dahl, R., 2007, *The BFG*, Puffin

Gersie, A. & King, N., 1990, *Storymaking in Education and Therapy*, Jessica Kingsley Publishers

Hughes, T., 1988, *Tales of the Early World*, Faber and Faber Ltd

Lipman, D., 1999, *Improving your Storytelling*, August House

O'Neill, C. & Lambert A., 1982, *Drama Structures – A Practical Handbook for Teachers*, Nelson Thornes

Pearson, J. (ed), 1996, *Discovering the Self Through Drama and Movement: The Sesame Approach*, Jessica Kingsley Publishers

Reed, A.W. 1994, *Aboriginal Stories*, Reed New Holland

Sherbourne, V., 1990, *Developmental Movement for Children*, CUP

Slade, P., 1995, *Child Play: Its importance for Human Development*, Jessica Kingsley Publishers Ltd.

For more information on Dramatherapy visit:

www.thedramatherapists.co.uk

www.badth.org.uk

www.sesame-institute.org

StoryBuilding

100+ Ideas for Developing Story & Narrative Skills

Sue Jennings

Improve literacy and communication skills & build confidence in narrative ability.

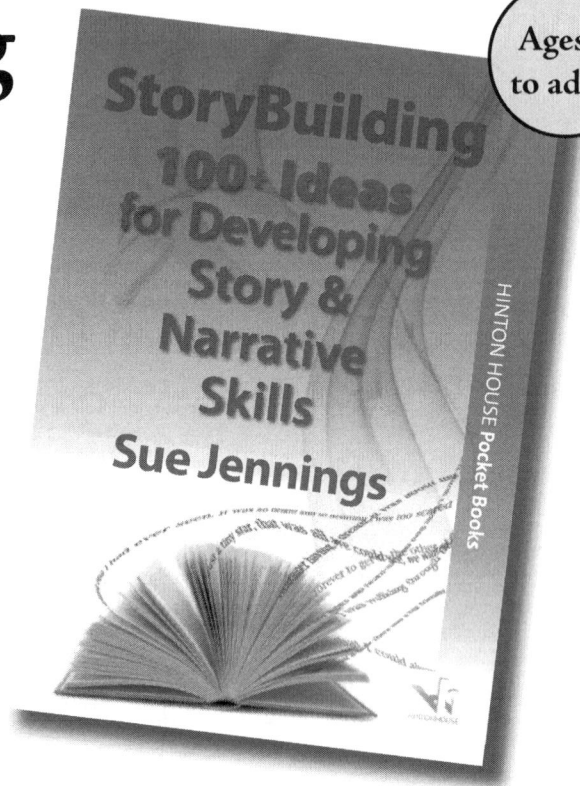

StoryBuilding
100+ Ideas
for Developing
Story &
Narrative
Skills
Sue Jennings

HINTON HOUSE Pocket Books

Ages 5 to adult

'StoryBuilding' will help young people understand the building blocks of a story and gain the confidence to create their own stories using the more than 100 themed story starters provided.

These are grouped developmentally and are accessible to young people of all ages and abilities. Each chapter contains themes and ideas for group discussions and homework suggestions. These will help youngsters to move from basic stories to more complex narratives. Story Starter worksheets provide templates for written story work.

Contents: Starting with 'Where?'; Starting with 'What Happened?'; Starting with 'Who?'; Developing Characters; Developing the Atmosphere; Developing the Props; Developing Places & Spaces; Starting with 'When?'; Developing the Plot; Endings.

2011 ◆ 120pp ◆ ISBN 978-1-906531-32-4

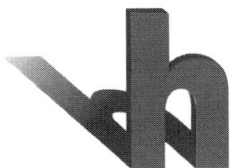

info@hintonpublishers.com • www.hintonpublishers.com